MECHANICAL SUTURES IN OPERATIONS ON THE ESOPHAGUS & GASTROESOPHAGEAL JUNCTION

MECHANICAL SUTURES IN OPERATIONS ON THE ESOPHAGUS & GASTROESOPHAGEAL JUNCTION

Felicien M. Steichen, M.D., F.A.C.S.
Professor of Surgery
New York Medical College
Valhalla, New York

Ruth A. Wolsch, R.N., B.S.

Published by: Ciné-Med, Inc.
127 Main Street North
Woodbury, CT 06798

ISBN: 0-9749358-6-7

Medical Illustrators:
William Baker
Robin Lazarus
Brooks Hart

Printed in Canada

TABLE OF CONTENTS

MECHANICAL SUTURES IN OPERATIONS ON THE ESOPHAGUS

Stapling instruments lend themselves particularly well to esophageal resection and reconstruction because of their precision and the decrease in tissue trauma, which is associated with the manipulation required to place multiple sutures. This is an important consideration in this fragile organ. Staples can be accurately placed in areas of narrow access such as the apex of the thorax and the base of the neck. The various anastomoses can be accomplished in a remarkable variety of ways with the linear anastomosing and closing techniques or with the circular anastomosing instrument. A particular advantage of the instruments used to perform anastomoses to the intrathoracic esophagus is that the remaining esophagus can essentially be left in its bed for the anastomosis, reducing the risk of disrupting its vascular supply by the mobilization usually required for placement of manual sutures. Mucosa-to-mucosa healing of the stapled terminal esophagus is as successful as that of other segments of the gastrointestinal tract, and the various anastomotic techniques shown have all been performed with satisfaction. Before the circular anastomosing instrument was available, we (Steichen, 1971; Ravitch, Steichen, 1972) and others (Chassin, 1978) have used the linear anastomosing and closing instruments for esophageal resection and reconstruction. There has been a flood of publications regarding the use of the circular anastomosing stapler, presumably because the inverting anastomosis it produces does not challenge accepted surgical doctrine like the linear anastomosing and closing instruments had. Another explanation for the excitement with which the circular anastomosing instrument was received lies in the fact that, although the use of mechanical sutures is reliably associated with greater ease and efficiency compared with manual techniques in the execution of a given operation, mechanical circular anastomoses are decidedly safer than all other anastomoses in the esophagus and rectum. At times, they enable the surgeon to perform an operation that could not have safely been done manually. Nevertheless, other stapling techniques, and of course manual anastomoses, continue to have a place in operations on the esophagus. As experience with the circular anastomosing instrument accumulates, it becomes increasingly apparent that some of the earlier difficulties with it resulted from attempting to force too large a cartridge into a narrow esophagus. The 31 mm cartridge is too large for the esophagus in most patients. Fekete and colleagues (Fekete, Breil, Ronsse, 1980; Fekete, Breil, Ronsse, Tossen, Langonnet, 1981) have pointed out the benefit of gentle progressive dilation of the esophagus with bougies or Hegar dilators before attempting insertion of the circular anastomosing instrument.

MECHANICAL SUTURES IN OPERATIONS ON THE CERVICAL AND THORACIC ESOPHAGUS BY CERVICOTOMY, THORACOTOMY, AND LAPAROTOMY

Cancer represents the most frequent indication for a thoracic esophagectomy, through a right or left thoracic or transhiatal approach (open or videoendoscopically), with preparation of the substitute organ through a separate laparotomy, and anastomosis to the cervicothoracic esophageal stump above or below the clavicles. In more rare cases, severe caustic burns, trauma, and other unusual conditions require a major esophageal procedure. Occasionally, only a substitute organ is necessary to bridge a congenital condition, in which case we prefer a carefully tailored left or, alternatively, right colon segment in an isoperistaltic mode. We have no experience with jejunal segments on a vascular pedicle in mid- or upper-thoracic locations and, in fact, have never been in the position where this technique would have represented the only solution. Similarly, we have never been associated with the use of free jejunal grafts in the neck. In the few cases where this substitute organ entered into the therapeutic choices, we have preferred the technically simpler, sturdier, and faster reverse duodenogastric tube, which still poses no small feat. In the five patients in whom this replacement was used after laryngopharyngoesophagectomy, we could not find a clear tumor-free margin above the mediastinal inlet to anastomose to a free jejunal graft. This was a clear indication to pursue the cervicomediastinal and transhiatal esophageal dissection, which is always easy with an anatomically normal thoracic esophagus. For comparison's sake, it can be argued that the blood supply of a gastric tube—even from a more distant origin—is as reliable as that of the free graft. In addition, the duodenum of the duodenogastric tube is wide, with an intact circular rim, and lends itself better to the pharyngeal anastomosis. If an anastomotic stricture occurs, there is only one proximal, accessible location with a gastroduodenal tube. There are two possible locations with a free jejunal graft.

ZENKER'S DIVERTICULECTOMY

Payne and Hoehn (Hoehn, Payne, 1969) from the Mayo Clinic reported their initial experience with four TA instrument closures of the neck of Zenker's pharyngeal diverticula. Payne and Reynolds (1982), with a clinical experience, since January 1, 1944, of 888 patients undergoing one-stage pharyngoesophageal diverticulectomy, stated, "During the past decade, we have utilized the TA 30 stapling device to effect closure and prefer it in terms of both speed and accuracy of closure." We have amputated 14 Zenker's diverticula at the University of Pittsburgh with the TA 30 or TA 55 instruments (Webster, 1982) with no leaks, fistulas, or strictures.

Following the initial report of Read from Little Rock, Arkansas, in 1970, epiphrenic diverticula have been amputated in the same way.

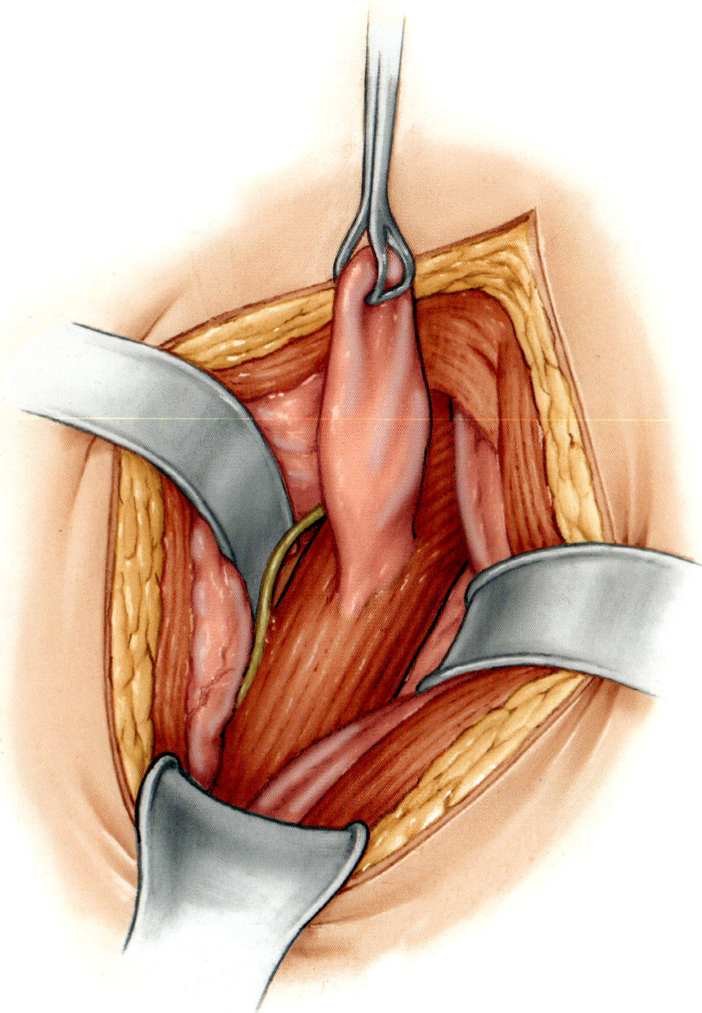

Figure III-1,A: A large tube or bougie is placed into the esophagus transorally, and the diverticulum is dissected through a left oblique neck incision and is gently elevated. As with all hollow viscera, one should avoid stapling a structure that is stretched by excessive traction.

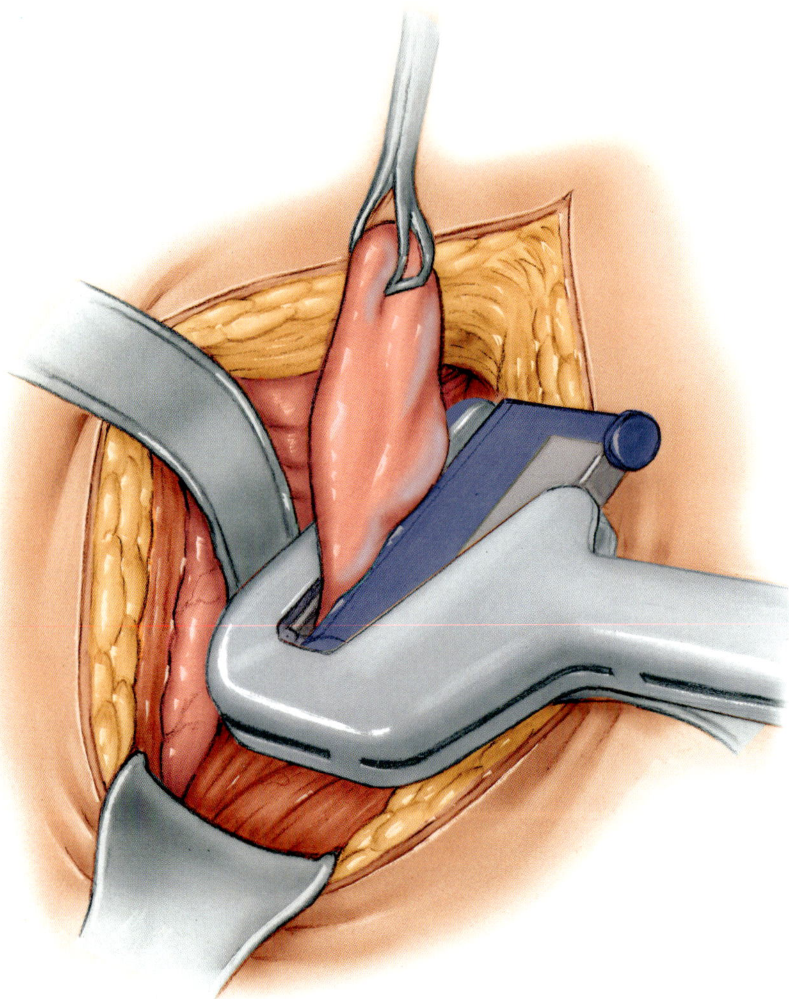

Figure III-1,B: The neck of the diverticulum is stapled with the TA 30 or TA 55/60 instrument so that the staple line will be parallel to the long axis of the esophagus, which usually is the longer dimension of the opening into the diverticulum from the pharynx. Payne and colleagues (Hoehn and Payne, 1969; Payne and Reynolds, 1982) prefer to apply it transversely. It may require a little manipulation to seat the TA 55/60 instrument in those patients in whom the neck of the diverticulum is too large for the TA 30 instrument. As always, the TA instrument is brought down to the tissue to be stapled—the tissue is not pulled up into the instrument. Following placement of the staples, the diverticulum is resected using the instrument's free edge as a guide for this transection.

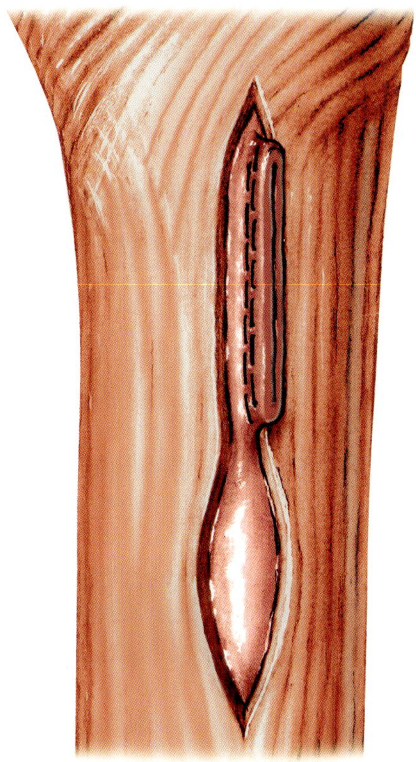

Figure III-1,C: The staple line requires no reinforcement (Payne [Hoehn, Payne, 1969; Payne, Reynolds, 1982] sutures muscles transversely over it). A myotomy, approximately 3 cm in length, is performed distal to and in continuity with the separation of the pharyngeal musculature, which was achieved previously by the pressure from the diverticulum.

REPAIR OF TRAUMATIC TRACHEOESOPHAGEAL FISTULA

Although a congenital tracheoesophageal (TE) fistula is a formidable challenge to the survival and hopeful longevity of the newborn, an acquired fistula, which fortunately is rare, is no less of a threat in the adult. If it is due to a malignancy, either from the tracheobronchial tree to the esophagus or vice versa, only a major bronchopulmonary and esophageal resection, with or without adjuvant therapy, and with esophageal replacement, will provide a chance of cure. It usually will result in palliation of bronchopulmonary aspiration and inanition and should therefore be undertaken only in patients who have sufficient physical and mental reserves to survive a very major surgical incursion and can expect to benefit from a prolonged quality-of-life improvement.

A TE fistula due to acute or insidious trauma is no less of a threat to survival than a congenital or acquired fistula. However, if recognized in time, it can be repaired with a perfect return to form and function of the two organs involved, as well as excellent survival of the patient. The more insidious occurrence due to repeated local insults from an endotracheal tube or a tracheostomy cannula in patients on prolonged artificial ventilation has practically been eliminated from our intensive care stations with the development of more safe and gentle intubation techniques and materials.

A massive acute fistula, resulting from the combined ill effect of the initial trauma and the necessity for speedy resuscitation in a patient with multiple injuries, can stretch the resources of an entire trauma team to its limits and exercise the ingenuity and skill of the surgeon and his or her team. By using the principle of double esophageal exclusion, proximal and distal to the repair, with linear staple lines placed across the wall and lumen of the esophagus and with the organ left in continuity (Figure III-10,A), Del Guercio successfully repaired a large complicated fistula in a young policewoman whose car had a disastrous encounter with a telephone pole during a high-speed chase. The patient had received initial care and had undergone a difficult endotracheal intubation at a local hospital. On arrival to the regional trauma center, the presence of multiple bilateral rib fractures, an increasing gastric air bubble in spite of a functioning nasogastric tube, and a continuous air leak through right-sided chest tubes (in the absence of any signs of abdominal trauma) pointed to severe intrathoracic injuries with an abnormal communication between the trachea and the esophagus and the right pleural space. After integrity of the aortic arch was established, an emergency right posterolateral thoracotomy was undertaken about 9 hours after injury.

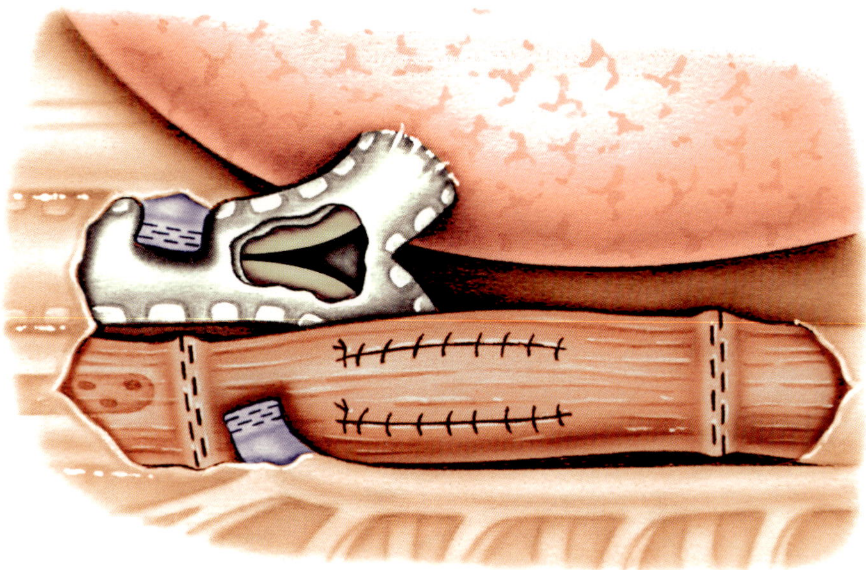

Figure III-2,A: Wide exposure of the mediastinum revealed a loss of substance of the membranous portion of the tracheal wall, just above the carina, and two 4 to 5 cm parallel lacerations of the anterior wall of the esophagus, with clean edges, starting distal to the lower border of the tracheal opening. Treatment required advancing the endotracheal tube into the right main bronchus and replacing it through its lumen with a smaller tube. A second tube was introduced alongside the existing tube and guided into the left main bronchus through the tracheal defect. Each endotracheal tube was connected to an individual respirator, allowing for separate inhalation anesthesia and ventilation postoperatively and for temporary pulmonary collapse of the right lung during repair. The clean longitudinal esophageal lacerations were repaired with individual manual sutures. The nasogastric tube was pulled to a level above these repairs, and the esophageal wall and lumen were closed transversely with TA 55-4.8 linear staple lines above and below the sutured lacerations. Suction on the proximal intraesophageal tube prevented the accumulation of saliva and nasopharyngeal secretions in the blind proximal esophagus. It also prevented fluid spillover through the intubated larynx into the tracheobronchial tree. The distal esophageal closure eliminated reflux of gastric acid secretions into the repaired esophagus, with corrosion of the suture lines.

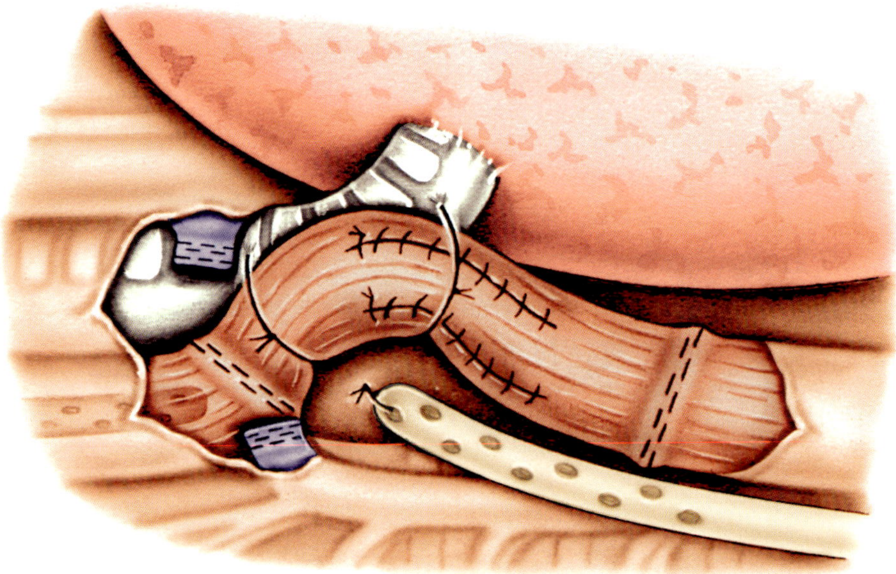

Figure III-2,B: The unstable chest wall, with many intercostal hematomas at the rib fracture sites, did not augur well for the raising of an intercostal muscle or even a simple pleural flap to cover the tracheal defect and act as a cushion between the esophagus and trachea. Since the esophagus was reliably repaired and excluded temporarily from swallowing and transport functions, its healthy portion proximal to the sutured lacerations was elevated and used as an onlay graft to cover the tracheal defect.

About 3 weeks later, after the patient had completely recovered, bronchoscopy and esophagoscopy demonstrated a normal-appearing tracheal mucosa without any stricture. The esophageal lumen was widely patent with minimal wall thickening at the transverse staple sites. Radiographic examination showed the staples in various stages of open B-configuration, embedded in the esophageal musculature.

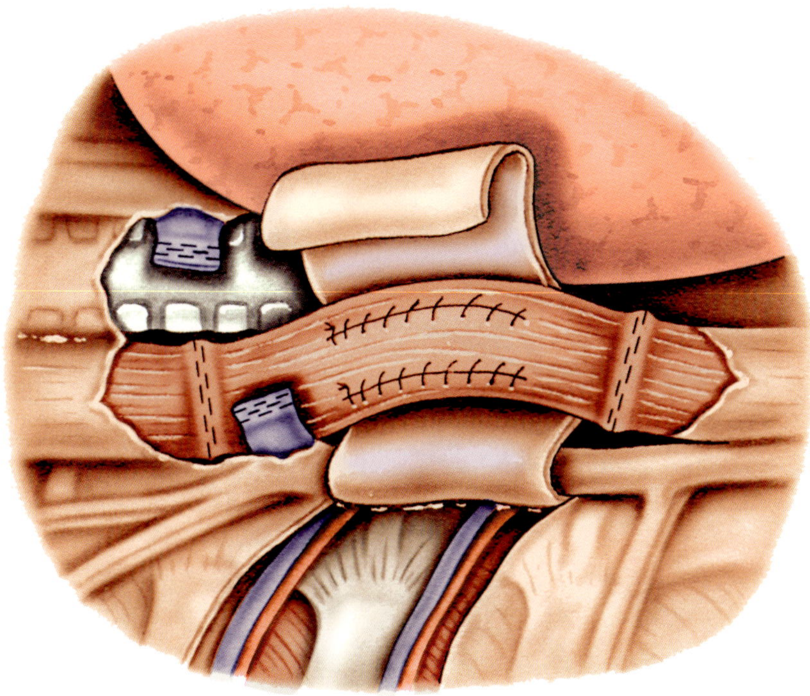

Figure III-2,C: In this patient, it did not seem wise to further compromise an unstable chest wall. We had to rely on a somewhat tenuous reconstruction, admittedly reinforced by the temporarily, functionally excluded esophagus. However, we would generally prefer to reinforce the repair of an injury of this magnitude with an interposed pleural flap.

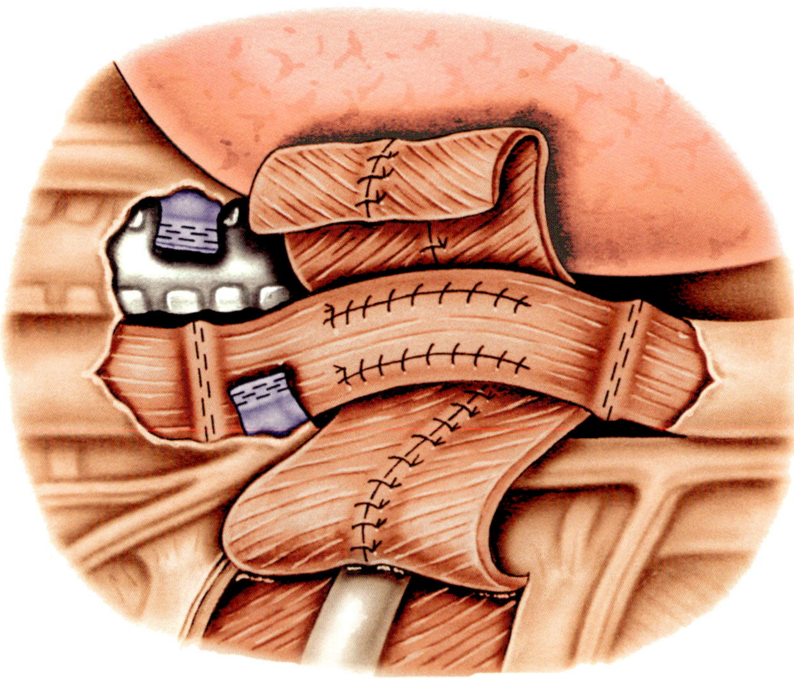

Figure III-2,D: Alternatively, the repair can be reinforced with two intercostal muscles, sutured together after removal of the rib in between.

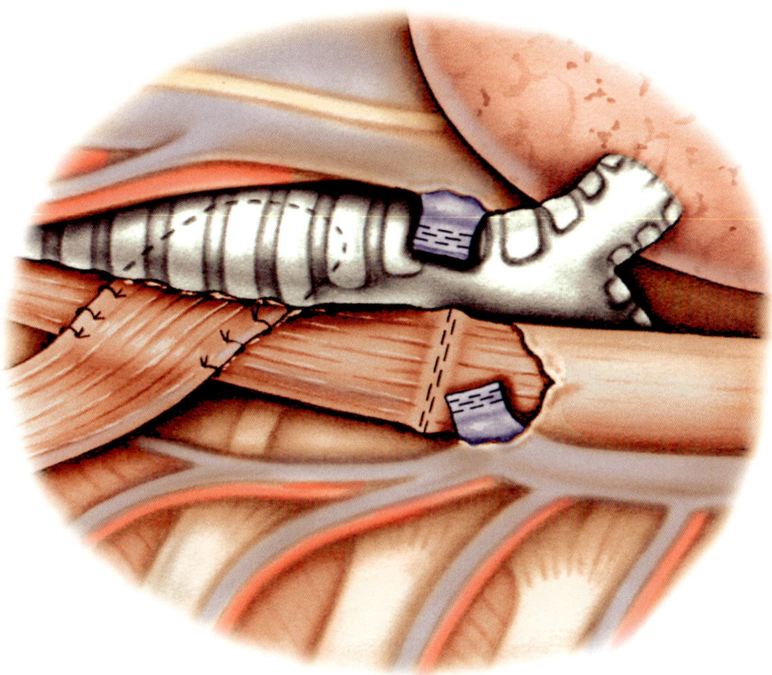

Figure III-2,E: In patients with a high TE fistula, a classic complication of a prolonged and difficult intubation, the repair can take place through a suprasternal cervical approach and a flat intact neck muscle can be sandwiched between the trachea and the esophagus. If acid reflux (not uncommon with mechanical ventilation) is to be avoided, the esophagus below the repair can be closed temporarily with an ENDO TA instrument through a right thoracoscopy.

ESOPHAGECTOMY AND REVERSE GASTRIC TUBE: GAVRILIU I

This operation is indicated in patients with cancer of the proximal half of the thoracic esophagus, without metastatic extension below the diaphragm. The procedure shown here is a Beck-Jianu-Gavriliu reverse gastric tube.

The indications for routine, simultaneous, or delayed one-sided or bilateral neck dissection in the absence of macroscopically recognizable lymph node metastases remain unresolved. Studies, mostly by Japanese authors, give validity to the concept of radical neck dissection in operable and hopefully curable cancers of the cervical and thoracic esophagus. It would appear, however, that one-stage radical esophagectomy, creation of a substitute organ, and classic or modified neck dissection(s) represent a formidable challenge for these often nutritionally compromised patients, as well as for one team or even several teams of surgeons.

The concept of sentinel node mapping and biopsy—so successfully used in operations for melanoma and breast cancer—may help in solving this dilemma. For an elongated organ such as the esophagus, spanning three anatomical spaces—the neck, mediastinum, and abdomen—and lacking the protective cover of a serosa, the lymphatic drainage can be unexpectedly erratic. Although the various patterns of drainage to the three potential lymph node basins are statistically well established for any tumor level, the knowledge that in a small number of patients all three locations are possible, could be interpreted as the need to radically excise all three lymphatic basins for any curative operative attempt—an almost impossible task in an operation as demanding as is the excision and replacement of the esophagus. Therefore, the intraoperative detection, biopsy, and histological examination of sentinel nodes below the diaphragm and above the clavicles could be of great value in proving the absence or presence of metastatic disease. A clear upper abdominal lymphatic basin would establish the performance of a reverse gastric tube on a secure basis. Clear or only unilaterally involved cervical lymphatic basins would justify the withholding of radical neck dissections or establish the approach on the side of identified metastatic disease for both the lymph node dissection and the esophago-substitute anastomosis. Since the thoracic esophagus is always excised—either by thoracotomy or thoracoscopy—a complete dissection of fatty and fibrous tissues in the posterior mediastinum, around the trachea, main bronchi, pericardium, and pulmonary vessels and aorta, on the side exposed by the approach, should be part of the excision, as far as the density of vital organs in this area allows an "en bloc" dissection.

The reverse gastric tube has a rich and dependable blood supply, requires only a slender channel to pass through in either substernal or posterior mediastinal position, and readily reaches the neck. The staple-constructed gastric tube transports food efficiently and empties readily into the stomach.

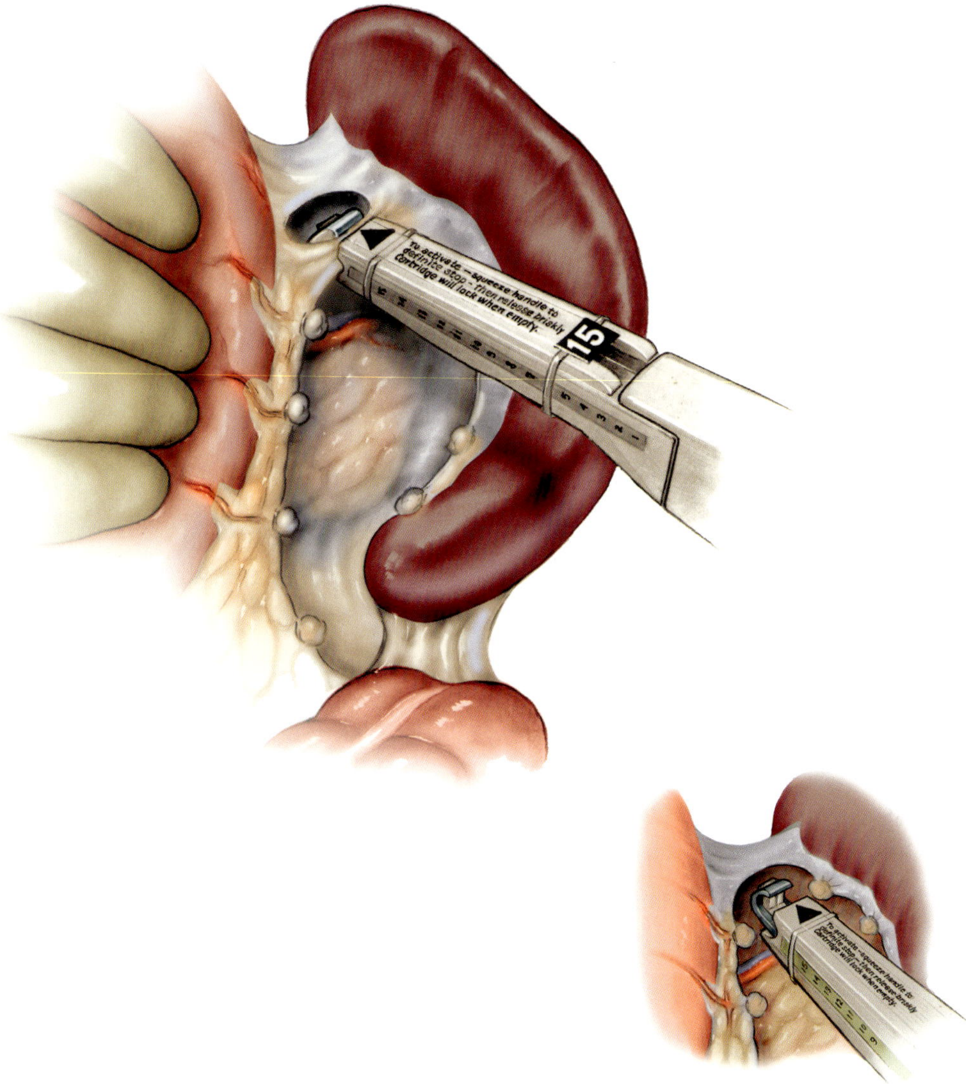

Figure III-3,A,B: The pertinent vascular anatomy is demonstrated. The gastroepiploic vessels are not always as beautifully continuous as they are shown, and, in fact, there usually is a gap high up on the fundus, bridged by reliable intramural vascular connections. While taking care to protect the left gastroepiploic arcade, the short gastric vessels are ligated and divided, either manually or with the LDS stapling instrument, close to their origin from the splenic vessels, following incision of and exposure through the gastrosplenic ligament. When activated, the LDS instrument places two crescent-shaped staples, ligating the tissue held within the jaw of the instrument, and evenly cuts between them.

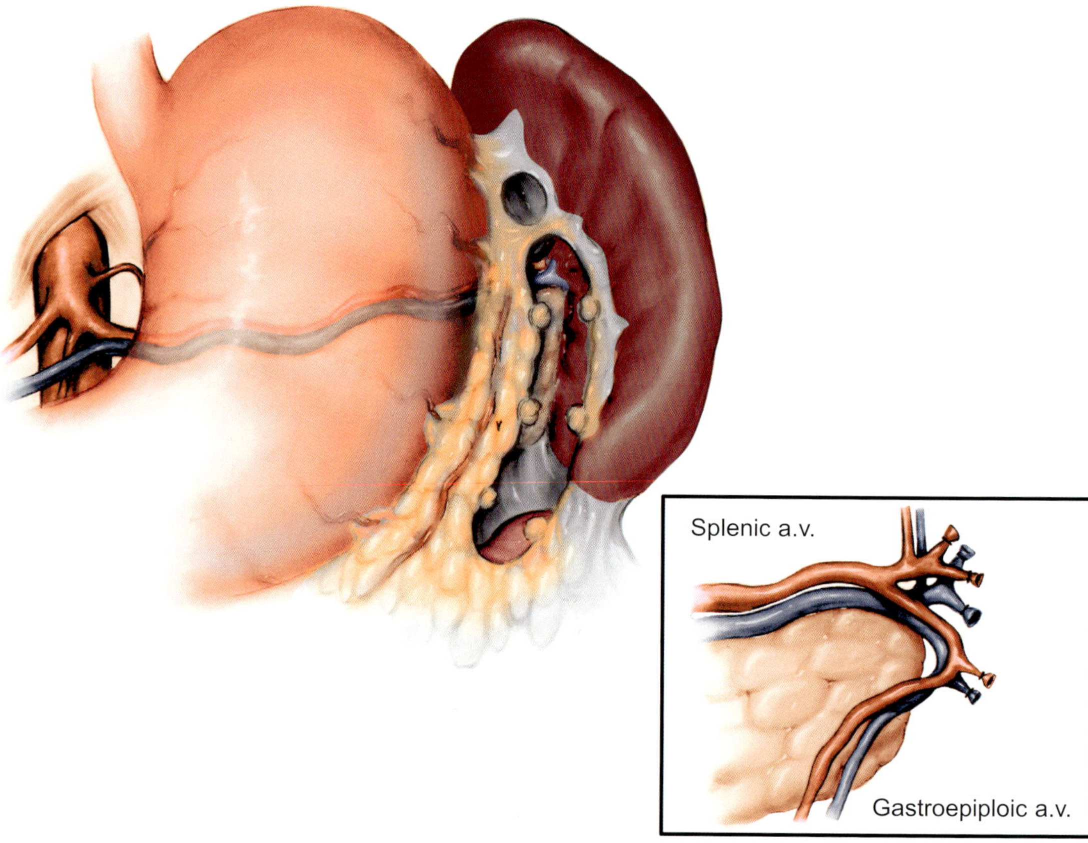

Figure III-3,C,D: In the adult, splenectomy is usually required to facilitate the development of a tube long enough to reach the desired level at the cervical esophagus or hypopharynx. The tube is based on the left gastroepiploic vessels, originating from the splenic artery and vein. However, we make a reasonable effort (in line with the length of gastric tube required) to preserve the spleen and, in fact, succeed in doing this in children, in whom preservation of the spleen is an immunologic sine qua non.

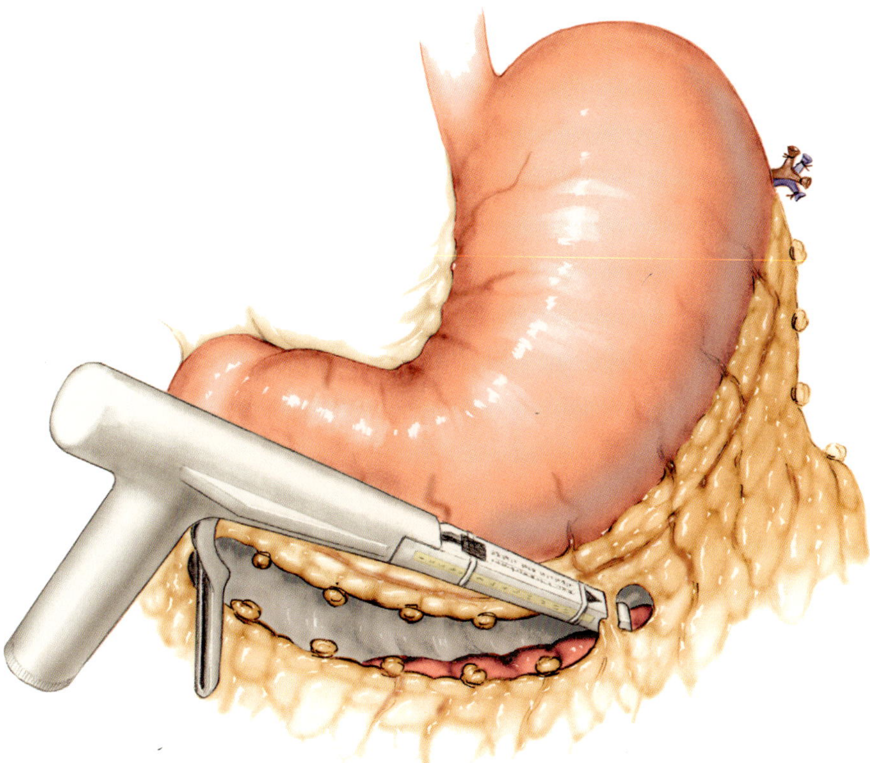

Figure III-3,E: The gastrocolic omentum is serially stapled and divided with the LDS instrument just peripheral to the gastroepiploic vessels. The right gastroepiploic vessels are divided at the level at which the tube is to be begun, peripheral to their origin from the gastroduodenal vessels.

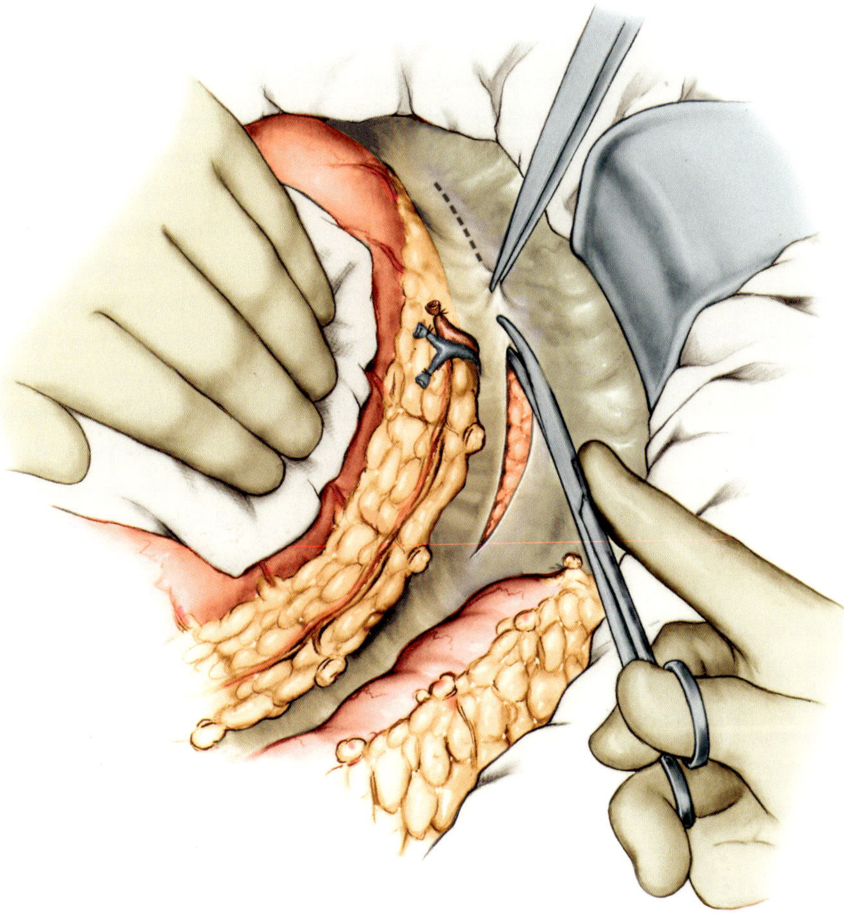

Figure III-3,F: The stomach is lifted forward, and the loose posterior peritoneal attachments are divided, exposing the tail of the pancreas. The pancreas is elevated from its retroperitoneal bed, in a medial direction, to the level of the aorta. This, together with the Kocher maneuver for the duodenum, gives great mobility to the entire gastric tube.

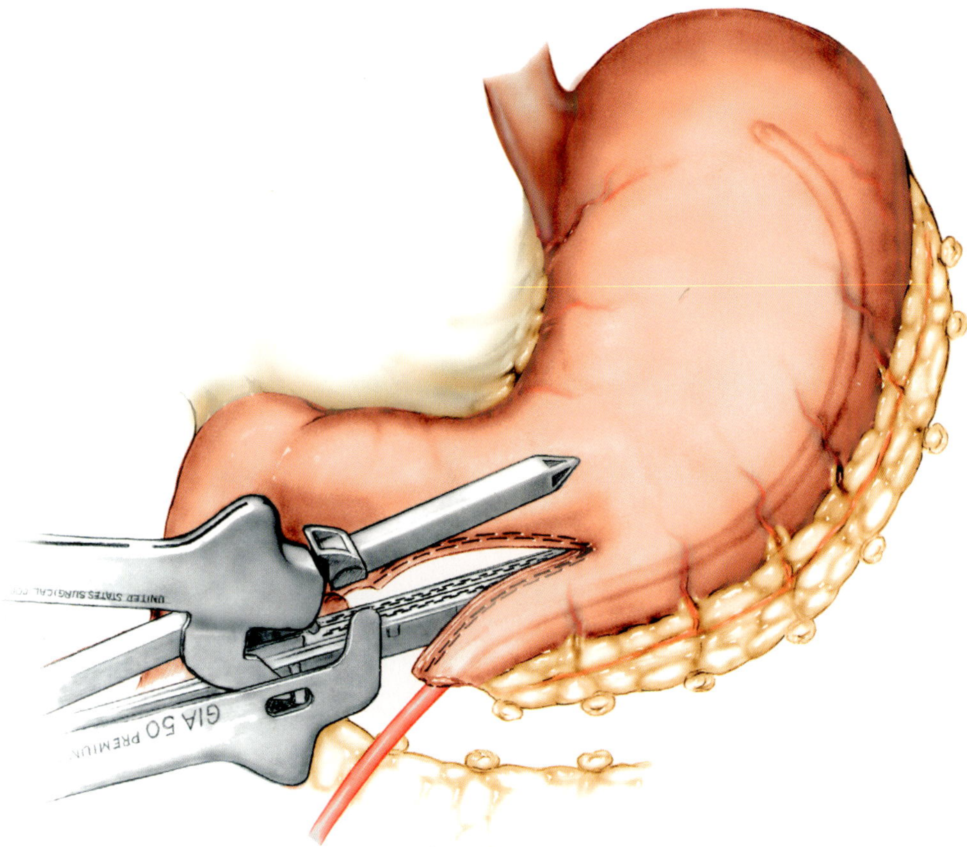

Figure III-3,G: A French #38-40 bougie is inserted into the stomach through a distal incision in the greater curvature approximately 2 cm proximal to the pylorus. The stomach is serially stapled and divided longitudinally along the edge of the bougie with repeated applications of the GIA instrument.

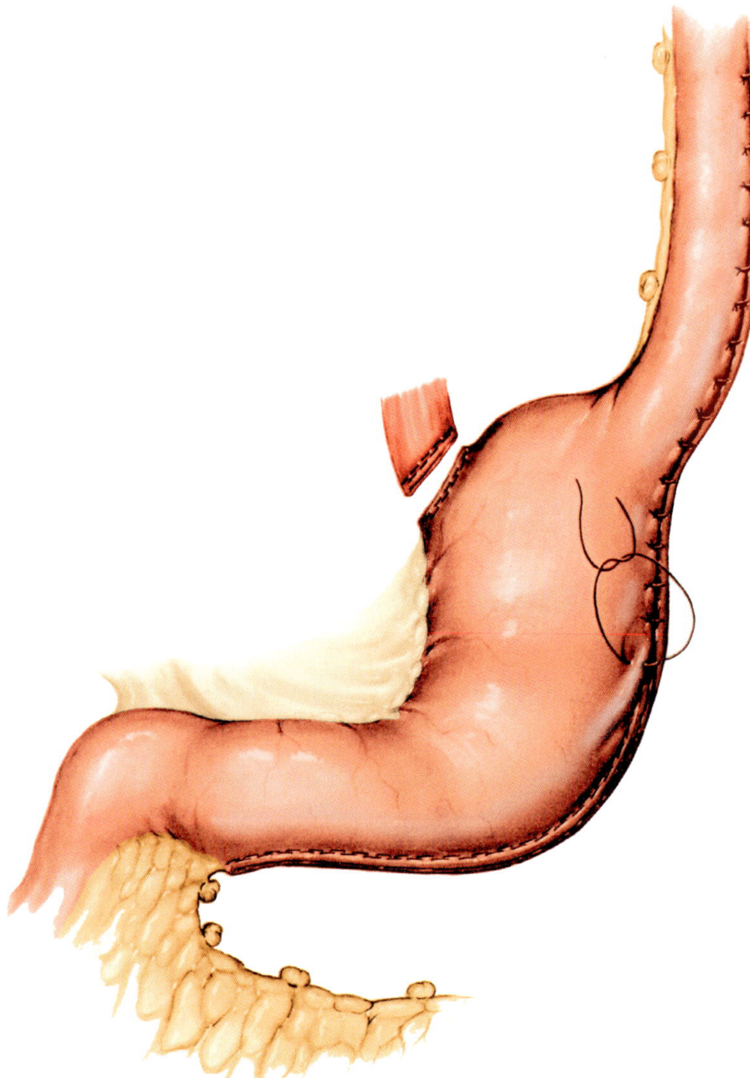

Figure III-3,H: Several applications quickly produce a tube that will easily reach above the clavicles. We oversew the GIA staple closure of the stomach and tube with a continuous suture or, if time permits, interrupted sutures (as shown) for hemostasis of thick gastric walls. This also avoids overstretching the tube and creating gaps between individual staples as the tube is elevated into the neck or apex of the chest. Toward the upper end of the tube, a continuous oversewing suture is replaced by interrupted sutures so that it is not divided if the tube requires shortening, or is anastomosed to the cervical esophagus with the circular instrument. If esophagectomy is part of the operation, the esophagus is divided from the stomach with the GIA instrument. Early on in our experience with this procedure, we routinely added a pyloroplasty. However, it soon became evident that this was not a mandatory step and that the pylorus relaxed and emptied readily after a short postoperative period of hesitation.

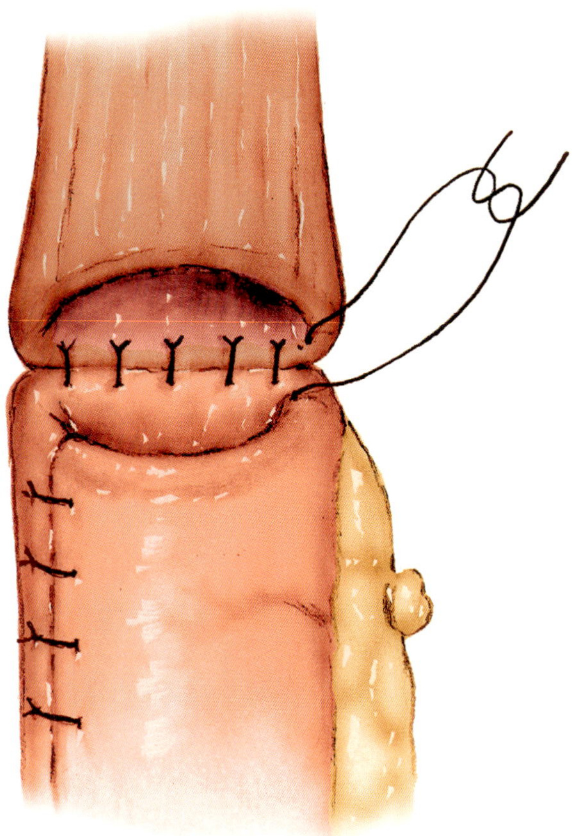

Figure III-3,I: If the gastric tube is to be placed into the original bed in the posterior mediastinum, it is attached to the abdominal segment of the esophagus following liberation of the esophagus in the chest and neck. The esophageal specimen is then pulled out through the neck incision, and the gastric tube follows the upward movement without twists and undue resistance. Care is taken to maintain the blood supply on the left side of the gastric tube, which means that the long staple and suture line will gently rotate to the right side into the neck. The anastomosis of the tube to the hypopharyngeal and/or cervical esophageal stump can be achieved manually, in one layer, with full-thickness interrupted sutures as shown here, or with a posterior running suture and anterior interrupted sutures.

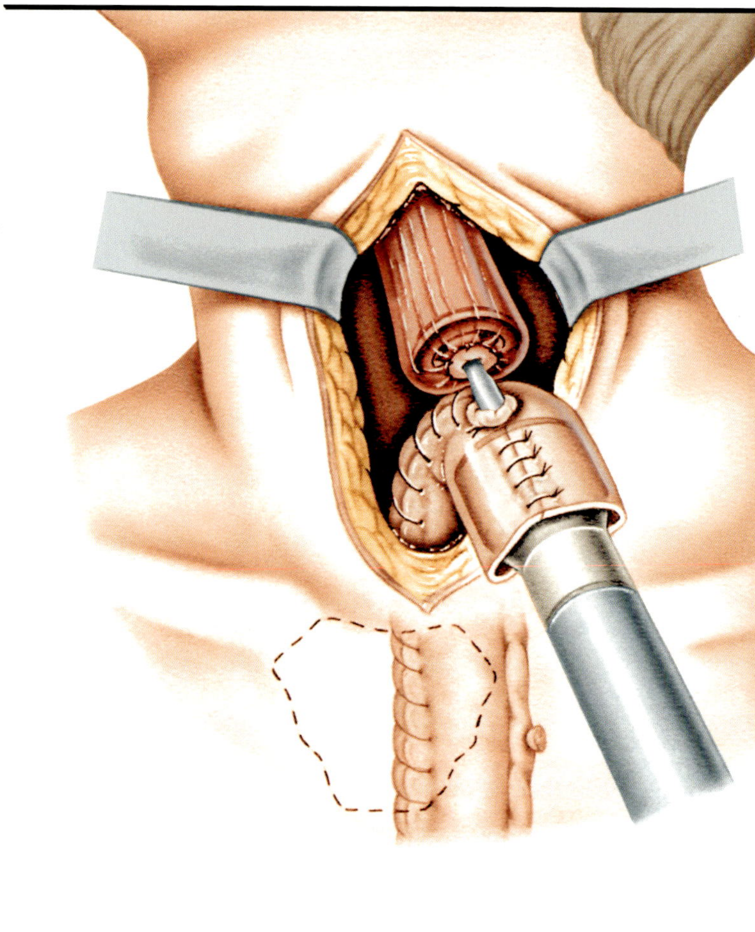

Figure III-3,J: If the gastric tube is of sufficient length, a stapled circular anastomosis can be performed through the open end of the gastric tube as an end-to-side esophagogastrostomy, functioning essentially as an end-to-end anastomosis. The anvil of the EEA instrument is advanced into the esophageal stump, and the previously placed purse-string suture is tightened around the anvil shaft. With the gastric tube shaped like the handle of a cane, the instrument cartridge is positioned into the open gastric tube lumen and the center rod is advanced through the staple line, 5 to 6 cm beyond the open tube lumen. A manual purse-string suture is placed around the perforation site and tied around the center rod to ensure that the tissue is held securely within the EEA instrument. The anvil shaft and center rod are joined, the instrument is closed and activated, and a double stapling (circular through linear staple lines) anastomosis is performed.

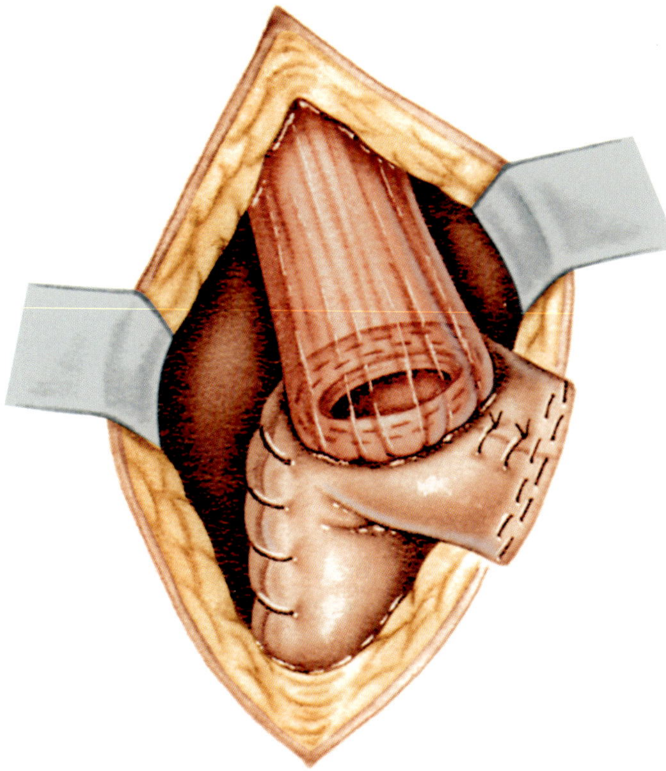

Figure III-3,K: After removal of the EEA instrument and inspection for hemostasis, the gastric tube is closed with a linear stapler and the excess tissue is resected along the edge of the instrument.

This type of anastomosis, as well as the manual one, is unfortunately associated with a definite incidence of strictures because of the shape of the anastomosis and the long lateral closure of the gastric tube.

LARYNGOPHARYNGOESOPHAGECTOMY AND EXTENDED REVERSE GASTRIC TUBE: GAVRILIU II

This operation is indicated in the treatment of cancer of the lower pharynx and cervical esophagus involving the larynx, as well as in tumors of the posterior larynx, extending into the pharynx and upper esophagus. If radical neck dissection is necessary and indicated, it may be performed by a second team while the reverse gastric tube is being prepared in the abdomen.

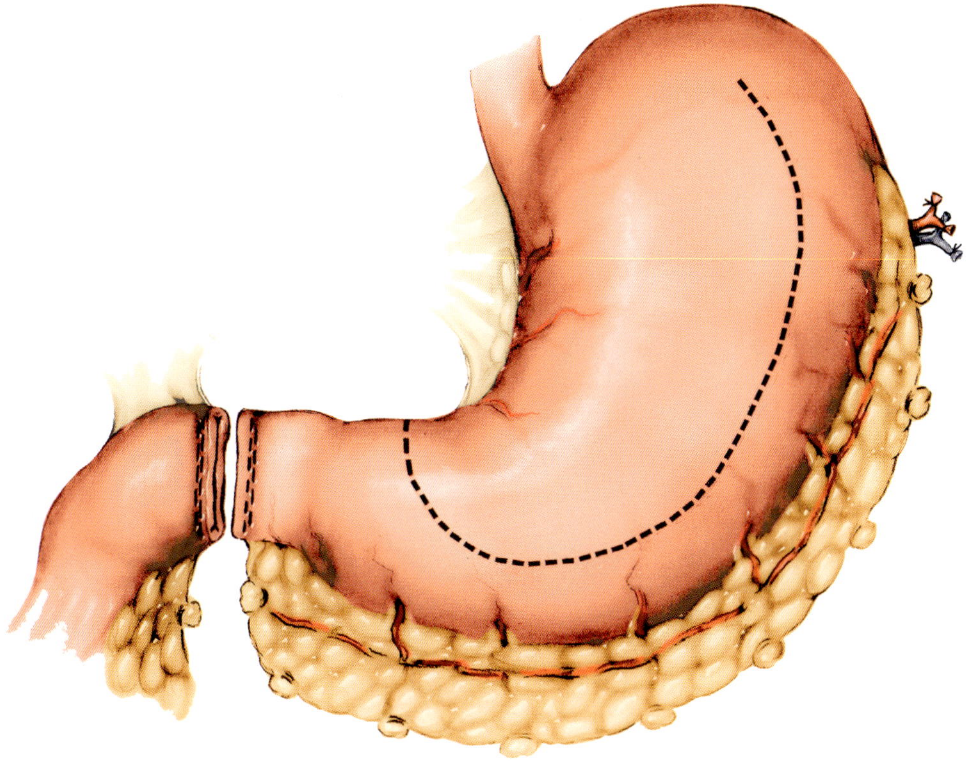

Figure III-4,A: Mobilization for this gastric tube is performed as described in Figure III-3, A to E, in continuity with an extension of about 2 to 3 cm beyond the pylorus. Since additional length is required for direct anastomosis of the gastric tube to the pharynx, the tube will follow the course shown by the dotted line, beginning on the lesser curvature (instead of the greater curvature) about 2 to 3 cm proximal to the pylorus. The duodenum has been stapled and divided by the GIA instrument at about the same distance beyond the pylorus. This step adds 4 to 6 cm to the length of the tube.

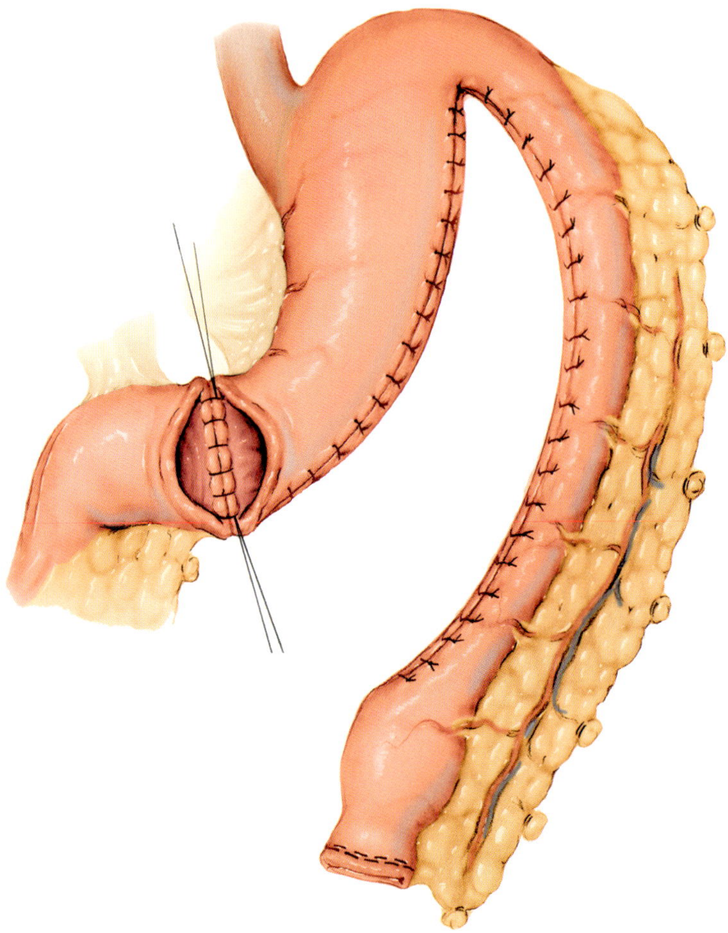

Figure III-4,B: The tube is shown completed. As in the Gavriliu I procedure, the staple closures of the stomach and tube are oversewn. The tubular gastric remnant along the lesser curvature is anastomosed manually to the duodenum after the GIA staple lines have been excised. As for the Gavriliu I reverse gastric tube, the left gastroepiploic vessels and the entire gastroepiploic arcade provide the vascular supply. To accomplish this vascular support, the right gastroepiploic vessels are divided behind the stomach, immediately beyond their origin from the gastroduodenal vessels.

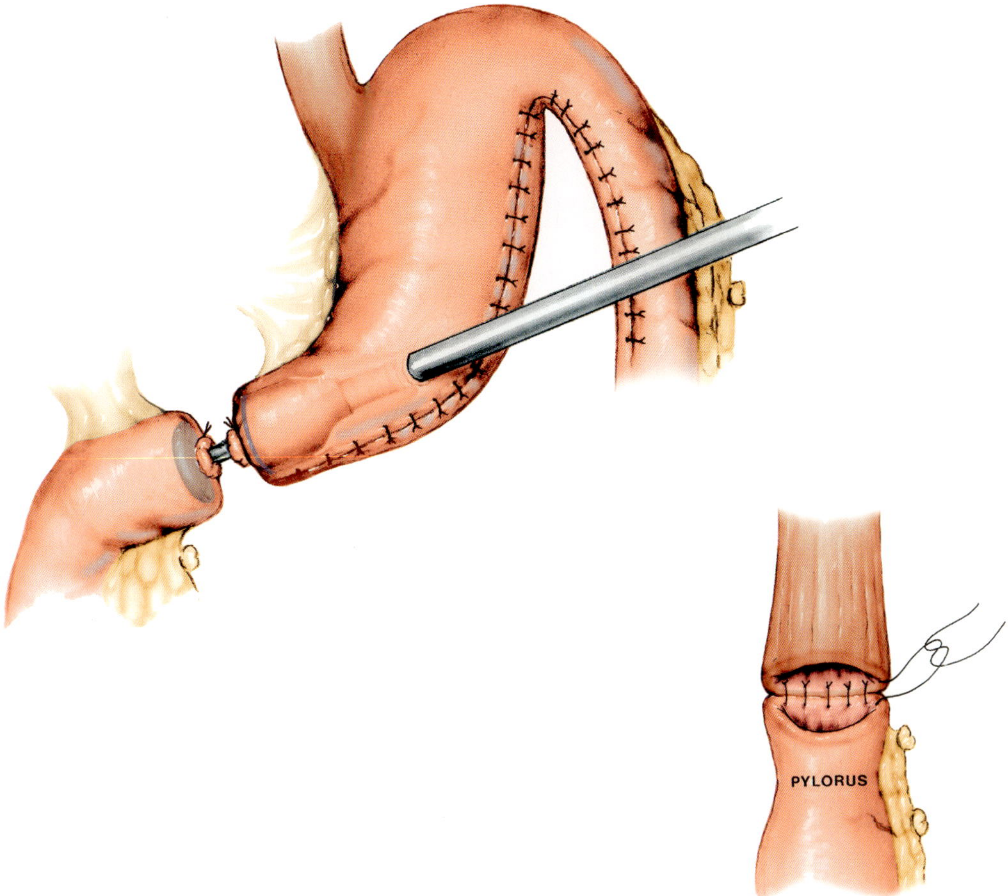

Figure III-4,C: Anastomosis of the gastric remnant to the duodenum can also be performed mechanically with an EEA instrument. The instrument, without anvil, is introduced through a proximal gastrotomy and positioned at the site for anastomosis. The center rod is advanced through the distal end of the remnant and a manual purse-string suture is placed and tied. The anvil is positioned separately into the purse-stringed duodenum and the suture secured. The anvil shaft and instrument center rod are mated, and the instrument is closed and activated. Following removal of the instrument and inspection of the anastomosis for hemostasis and the tissue "donuts" for continuity, the gastrotomy is closed transversely with a linear stapler.

Figure III-4,D: This extended reverse gastric tube can be elevated through the anterior or posterior mediastinum, as indicated by circumstances in each individual patient. It is anastomosed manually to the hypopharynx in an end-to-end fashion.

Since this anastomosis reaches the inferior limits of the base of the tongue anteriorly and the pharynx is attached to the prevertebral fascia posteriorly, it would be impossible to place a purse-string suture safely in order to use the circular stapler at this level. Furthermore, the full intact circumference of the duodenum lends itself with great ease to a one-layer manual anastomosis.

ESOPHAGEAL PREPARATION FOR MECHANICAL CIRCULAR ANASTOMOSIS

Methods of circular anvil placement into the esophagus vary with the proposed site of anastomosis, the length of the remaining esophageal stump, and the surgeon's preference. The methods shown here can be used at any level of the esophagus, but are most helpful in the thoracic cavity, where the posterior space for manipulating the anvil and its shaft is limited by the spine. The triple stapling technique (Figure III-5, H to K) is most reliable. It is especially useful in transhiatal anastomoses since, at more proximal levels, the necessary upward and downward movement of the anvil will meet resistance by the endotracheal tube in the narrow thoracic inlet and in the short cervicopharyngeal segment in the neck.

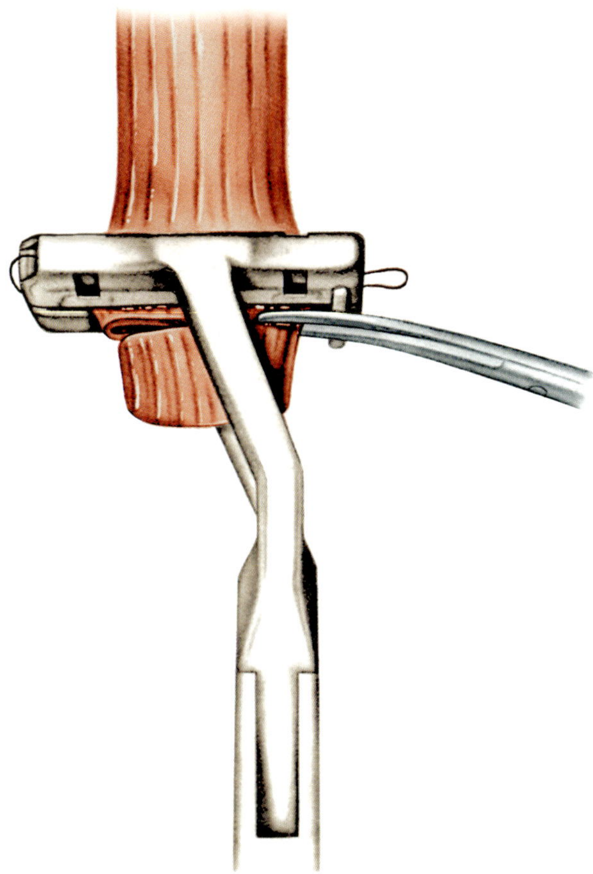

Figure III-5,A: Following removal of the specimen, the Purstring instrument is applied proximal to the resection and the excess esophagus is excised along the distal edge of the instrument. The purse-string suture can also be placed in an over-and-over whipstitch fashion by hand (Figure III-12,I) at the level of resection if the esophagus cannot be elevated sufficiently to apply the Purstring instrument.

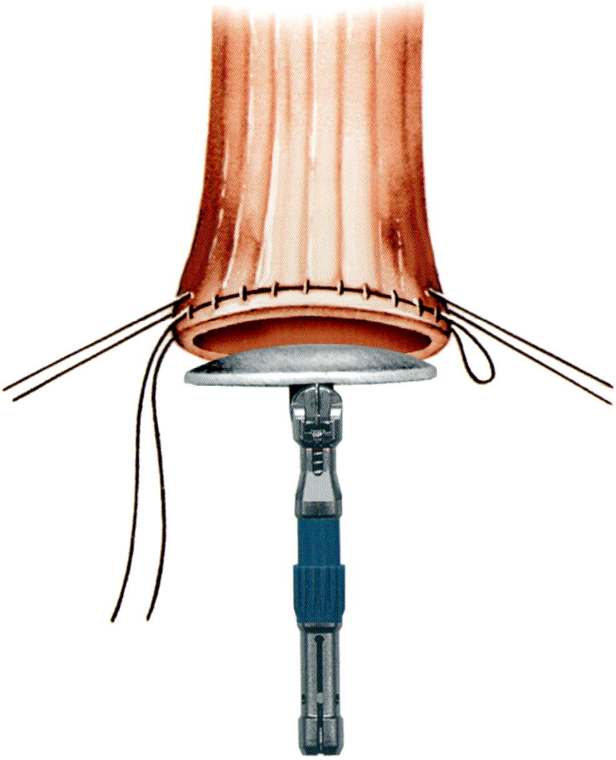

Figure III-5,B: The lumen of the esophagus is held open with stay sutures, and the anvil of the appropriate size EEA instrument is advanced into the previously dilated (Hegar dilators) esophagus. The purse-string suture is tied securely around the anvil shaft and is then brought around a second time in the tissue groove created by the circular tie, as shown in Figure III-5, D and G.

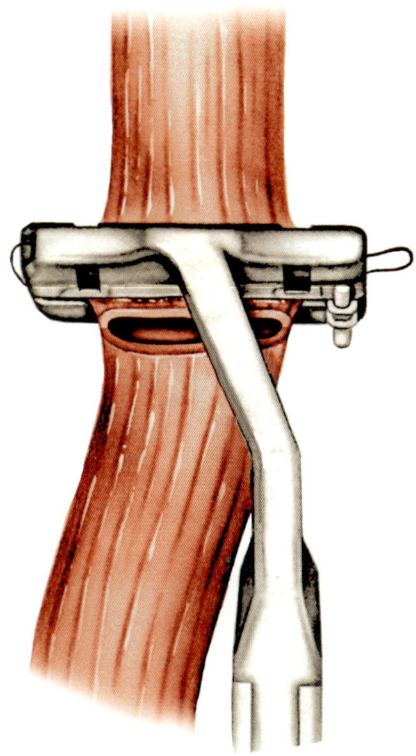

Figure III-5,C: A different technique will prevent retraction and maintain the esophagus clearly exposed in the operative site. In this scenario, the anvil is placed while leaving the specimen temporarily attached and using it to exert gentle traction. The Purstring instrument is applied at the planned level of resection and the anterior wall of the esophagus is incised, using the inferior instrument edge as a guide.

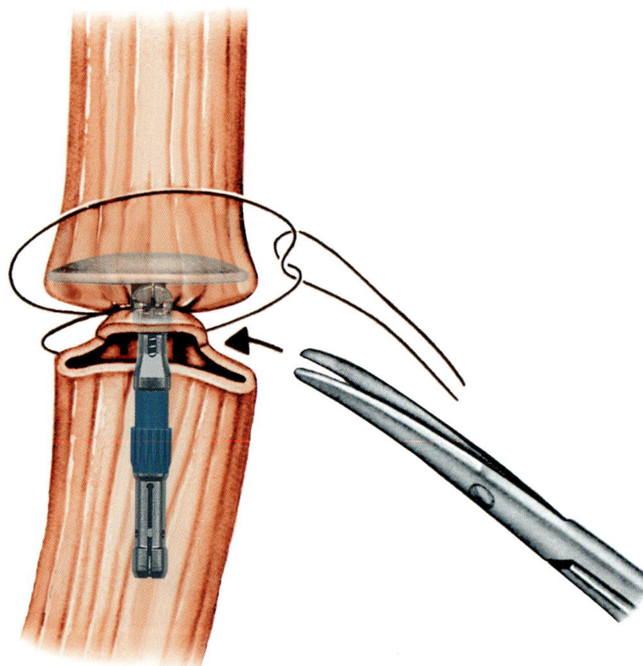

Figure III-5,D: Following removal of the Purstring instrument and placement of the anvil, the purse-string suture is tied and reinforced by a return sling and tie. Finally, the posterior wall of the esophagus is transected and the specimen removed. The reinforced purse-string suture is most reliable in securing the anvil and shaft within the muscular esophagus, short of the triple stapling technique, which is limited, however, to applications in the lower esophagus, well below the tracheal carina.

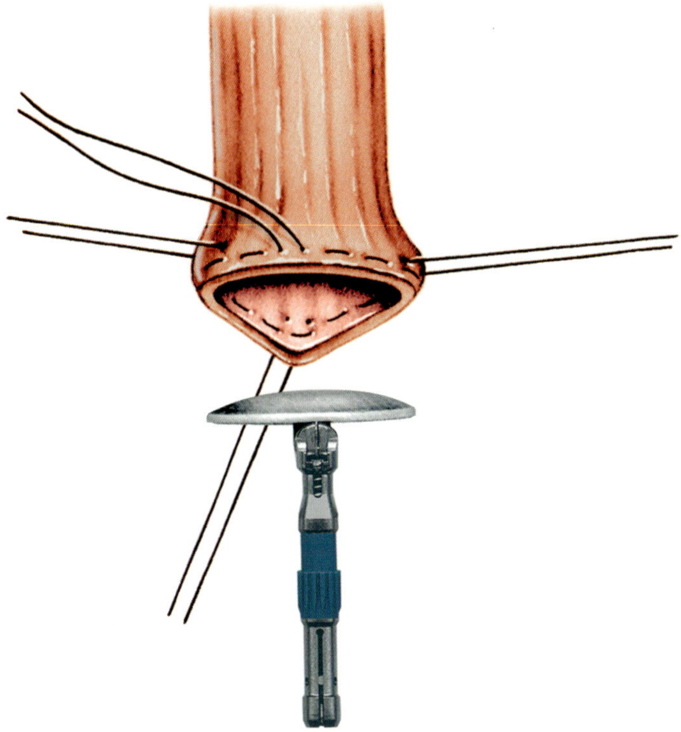

Figure III-5,E: Because of the deep location of the esophagus in anatomically crowded and narrow spaces, especially the neck and upper mediastinum, it may be difficult to establish satisfactory access into the esophageal lumen. The low profile shape of the anvil lends itself to the "tire-rim" mounting technique. The purse-string suture is introduced manually or mechanically, and three stay sutures are placed to hold the stationary esophageal circumference (the "tire") open. The mobile flat anvil (the "rim") is held vertically and advanced with half its circumference into the lumen of the esophagus.

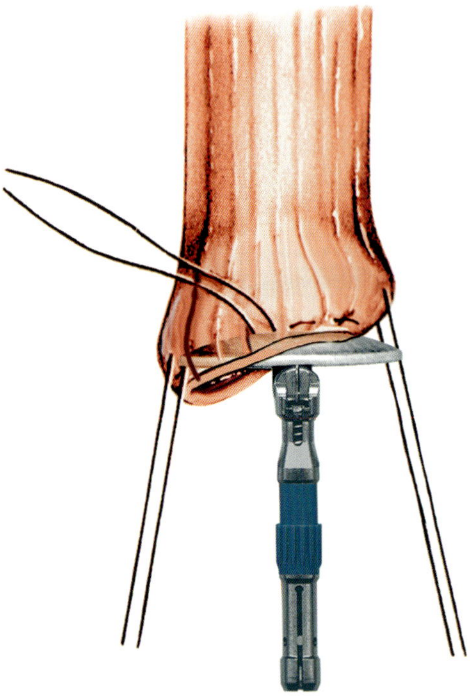

Figure III-5,F: While keeping gentle traction on the three stay sutures, the anterior circumference of the anvil (the "rim") is hooked behind the anterior esophageal ostium (the "tire") and with a pivoting downward movement of the anvil shaft, the entire anvil is securely placed within the esophagus.

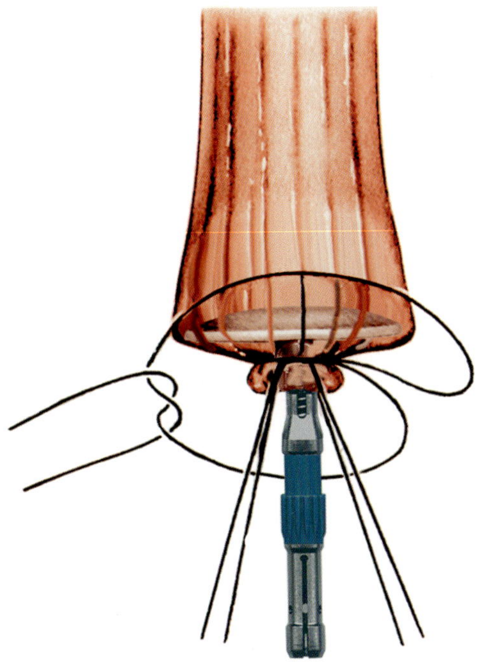

Figure III-5,G: The purse-string suture is tied securely and then reinforced with a second throw of the same thread.

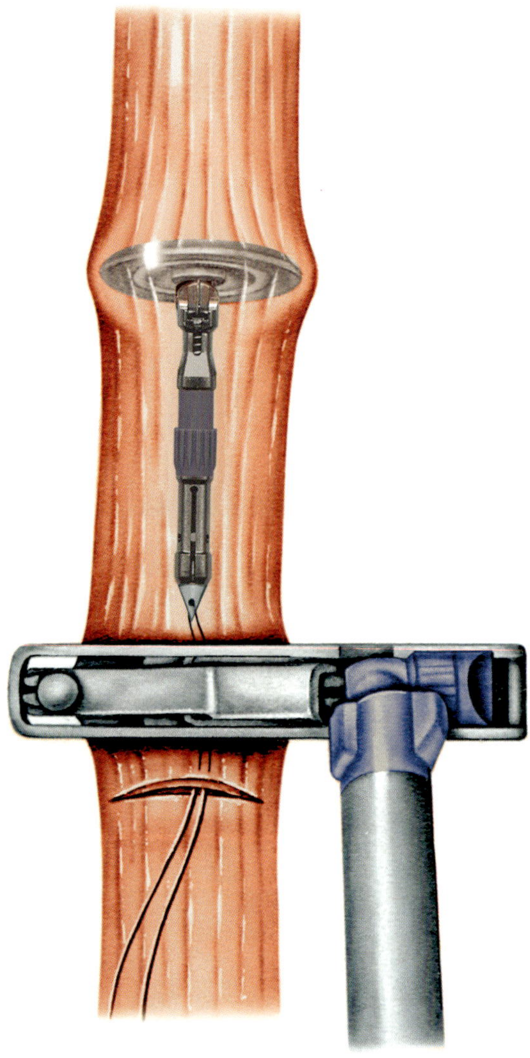

Figure III-5,H: For the triple stapling technique, a trocar tip, fitted with a heavy thread (leash) through the hole at its pointed tip, is attached to the anvil shaft. After irrigation and aspiration of the proximal lumen with occlusion of the esophagus just above the tumor (with a circumferential tape or thread not shown in these illustrations), the anvil is placed into the esophagus through a proximal anterior esophagotomy at a safe distance from the tumor. The anvil and anvil shaft are pushed proximally and held only by the leash let out through the center of the esophagotomy. The esophagus is closed just proximal to the temporary esophagotomy and distal to the trocar tip with the linear Roticulator stapler placed, in this case, through the enlarged diaphragmatic hiatus.

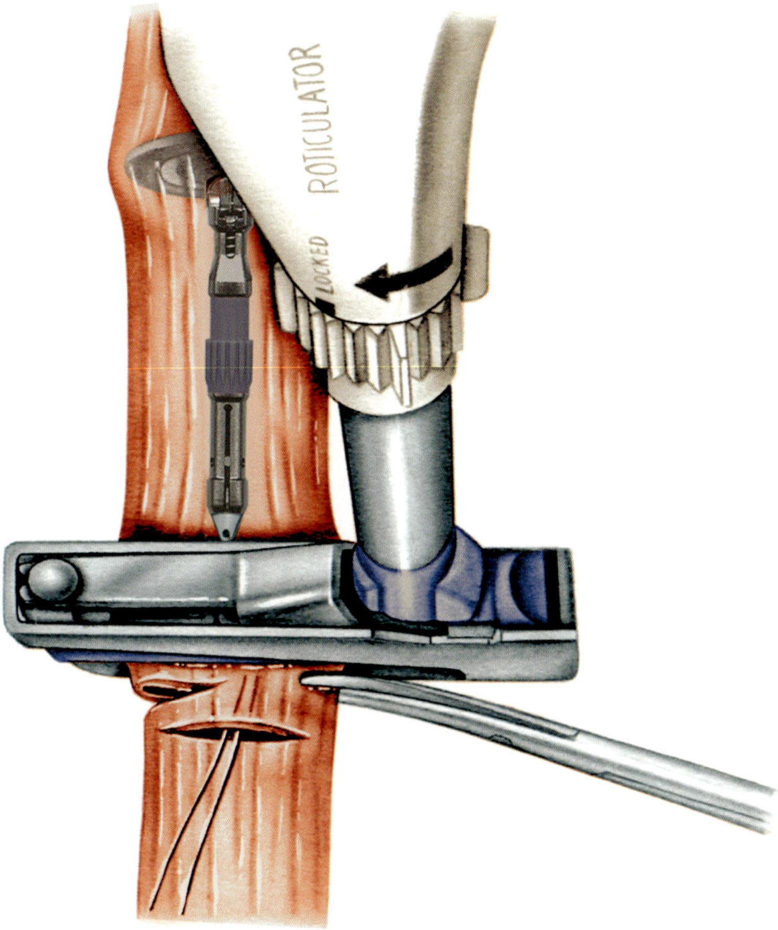

Figure III-5,I: The Roticulator instrument shaft is elevated to clear the approach to the esophagus, which is transected from both sides, taking great care to keep the leash intact.

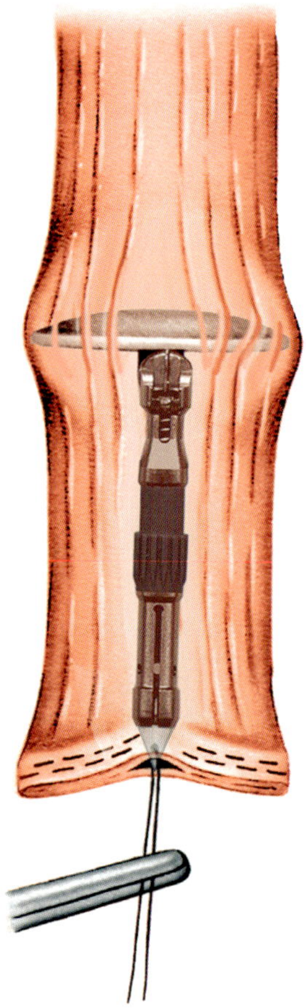

Figure III-5,J: The linear stapler is removed and the leash, followed by the anvil shaft, is pulled through the center of the linear stapled closure. The trocar tip is removed. The anterior gastrotomy is closed with a linear stapler.

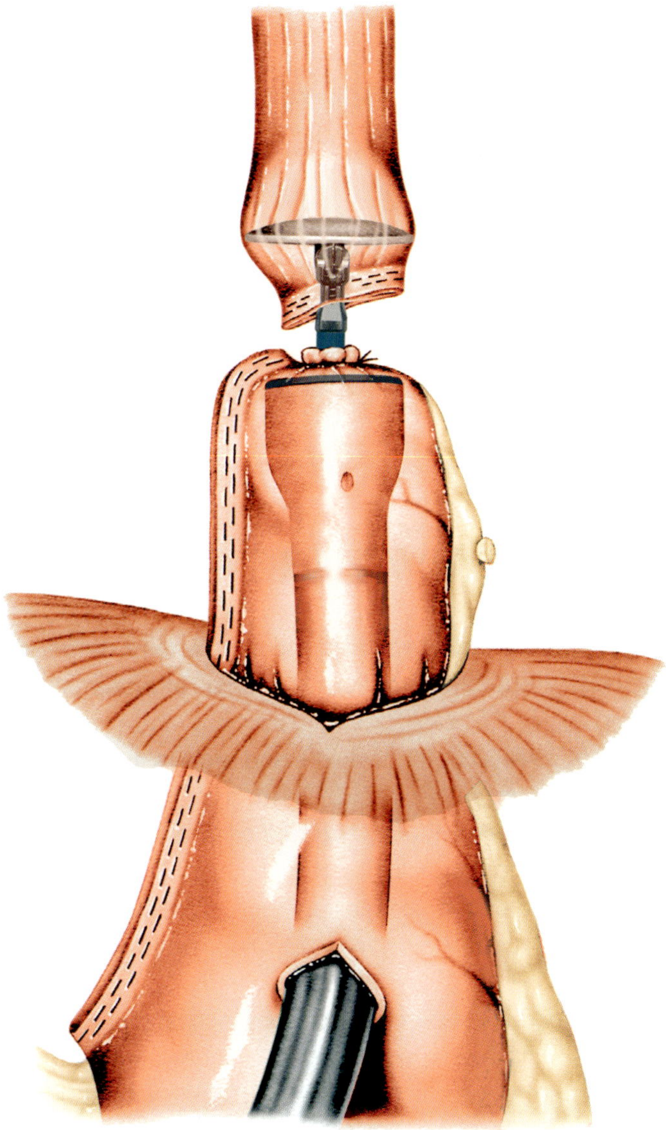

Figure III-5,K: In this case, the stomach, remaining after an esophagogastrectomy, is anastomosed to the lower esophagus transhiatally. The EEA instrument, without anvil, is introduced into the stomach through an anterior gastrotomy and positioned at the apex of the remaining stomach, near the linear closure of the fundus. The instrument is opened, advancing the center rod through the gastric wall. A manual purse-string suture is placed around the perforation site and tied around the center rod to ensure that the tissue is held securely within the EEA instrument. The entire assembly of stomach and instrument is guided into the posterior mediastinum from the abdomen. The anvil shaft and center rod are mated, and the instrument is closed, checked to make sure that no extraneous tissue is incorporated, and activated. The anastomosis is performed by an end-to-end circular stapling technique.

ESOPHAGOGASTRECTOMY AND ISOPERISTALTIC GREATER CURVATURE GASTRIC TUBE

This operation is useful in patients with cancer of the middle third of the esophagus. The need to obtain a safe margin caudally requires resection of a collar of proximal stomach, which makes a reverse gastric tube impossible. Excision of the lesser curvature elongates the stomach into a wide tube, based on the right gastroepiploic vessels and arcade that can be elevated into the base of the neck or the apex of the right or left chest. Under most circumstances, this is the preferred substitute for middle third lesions of the esophagus if an intact stomach is available; a modified version is used for lower third cancers. While it is technically simpler to construct, it has the disadvantage of elevating most of the gastric reservoir into the chest. A Kocher maneuver is performed on the duodenum in order to enhance upward mobility of the gastric tube.

While a radical mediastinal node dissection is indicated in all patients with a thoracic esophageal tumor, the pattern of lymph node drainage below the diaphragm and occasionally to the neck in middle and lower third lesions can be clearly established by sentinel node mapping, biopsy, and histological examination. In a potentially curative situation, the need for or abstention from an excision of the lesser omentum, and radical node clearing along the hepatic and splenic arteries, as well as the upper rim of the pancreas, can be clearly established by intraoperative definition of the histological character of the upper abdominal lymphatic basin, by using the sentinel node technique. Conceivably, as adjuvant therapies become more sophisticated, efficient, and target oriented in the future, it may be possible to use the sentinel node technique as a marker, remove the metastatic nodes identified by the node mapping, and leave the control of a possible early focus of microscopic metastatic disease, too small to be detected by the available node mapping techniques, to specific regimens of chemotherapy and/or radiotherapy.

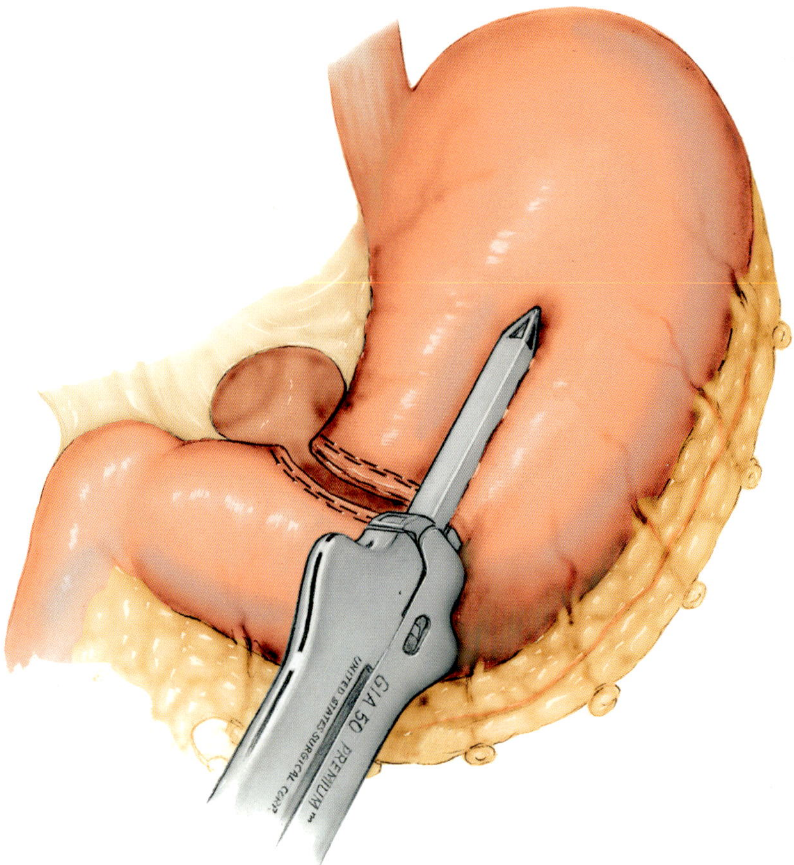

Figure III-6,A: The greater curvature of the stomach is mobilized, leaving the gastroepiploic vessels intact. The stomach is transformed into a wide, elongated tube by a marginal resection of the lesser curvature using serial applications of the GIA instrument, starting 2 to 3 cm proximal to the pylorus. The gastroesophageal (GE) junction and a collar of proximal stomach are part of this resection. The celiac axis lymph nodes are sampled and staged to confirm their negative status or to decide upon the extent of lymphadenectomy.

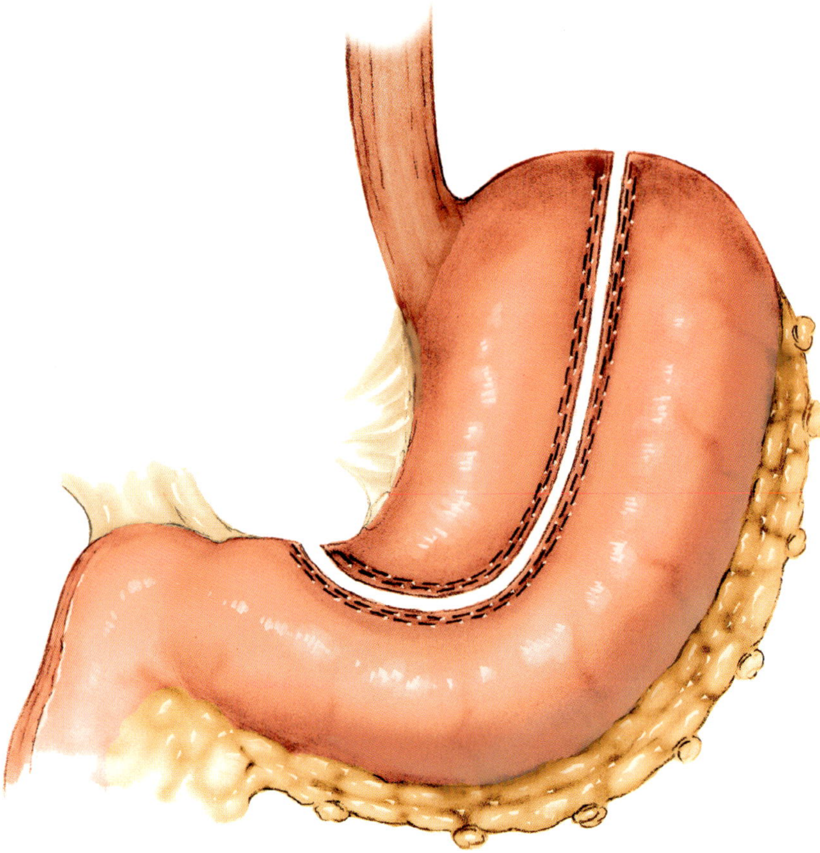

Figure III-6,B: The completed isoperistaltic tube and closed specimen are shown. The tube should be oversewn with a continuous suture or interrupted sutures.

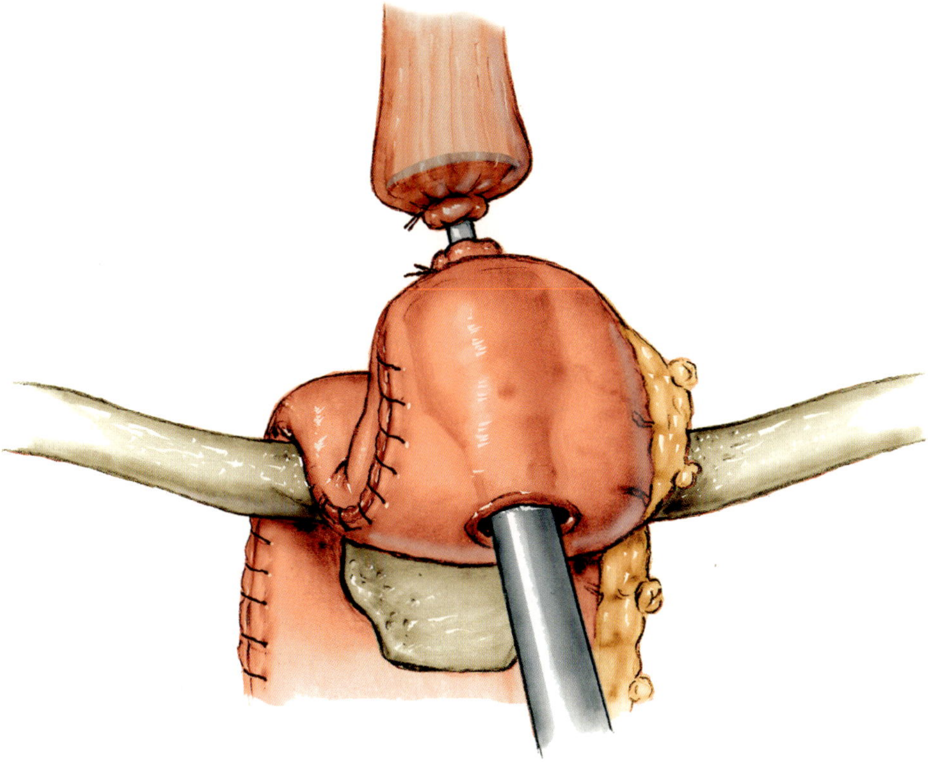

Figure III-6,C: The proximal end of the wide isoperistaltic tube is attached to the distal end of the specimen, and the previously liberated cervical and thoracic esophagus is pulled out through the left neck incision. The gastric tube is elevated into the neck in this fashion. If sufficient length is available, end-to-end esophagogastrostomy is possible with the circular stapling instrument placed through an anterior gastrotomy and the anvil advanced separately into the lumen of the esophagus—both are secured with purse-string sutures. The tissue is held snugly against the cartridge and anvil as the instrument is closed and checked to make sure that no extraneous tissue has been incorporated.

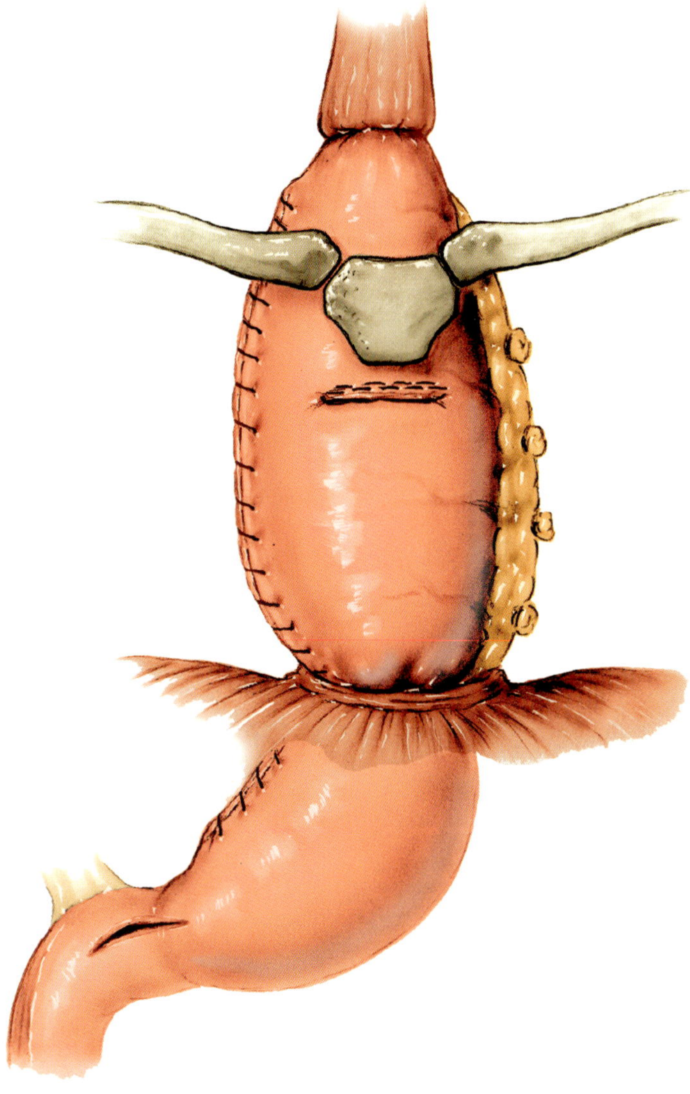

Figure III-6,D: The end-to-end anastomosis is between the esophagus and the fundus of the stomach. Following completion of the anastomosis, the circular stapling instrument is removed, the completeness of excised tissue "donuts" and integrity of the anastomosis are checked, and the anterior gastrotomy is closed with a linear stapler. The gastric tube is straightened by a gentle pull on the pylorus in the abdomen, which places the gastrotomy closure into the upper mediastinum.

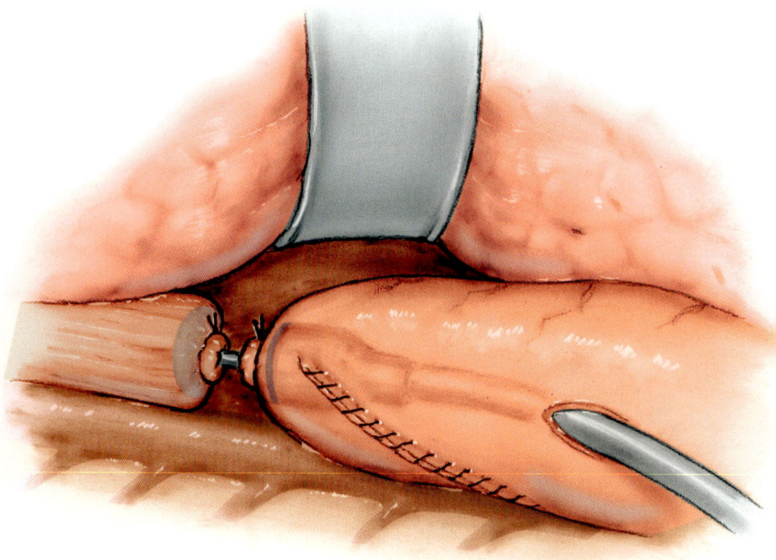

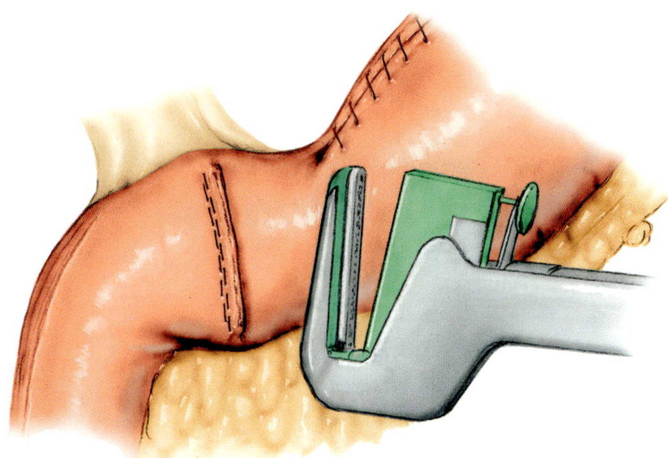

Figure III-6,E: If sufficient proximal esophagus remains, the esophagogastrostomy can be performed below the clavicle in the apex of the right chest cavity through a transthoracic approach.

Figure III-6,F: To facilitate evacuation of the stomach and limit retrograde pressure, a Heineke-Mikulicz pyloroplasty is performed using a linear stapler.

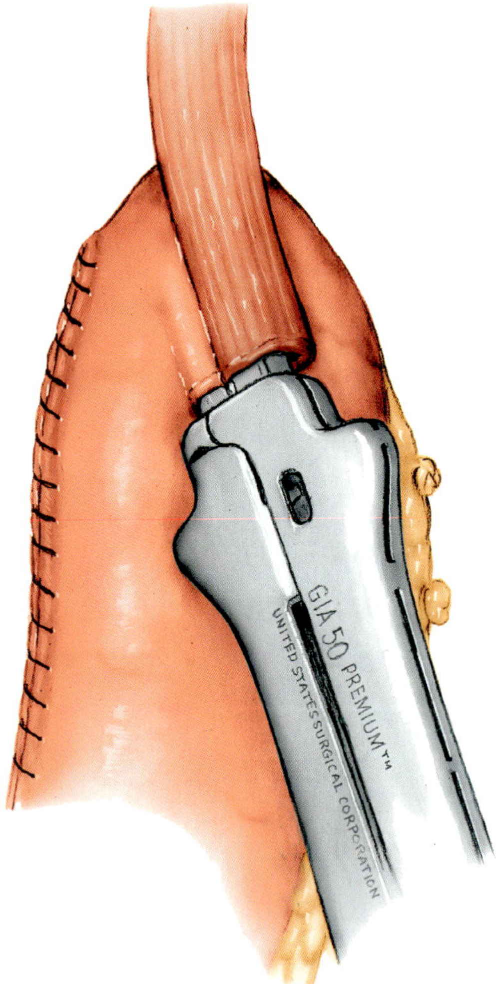

Figure III-6,G: If the esophagus is narrow and very muscular at the level of the proposed anastomosis and a circular stapling instrument of sufficient caliber to avoid stenosis (28 mm) cannot be used, then a linear, true side-to-side or functional end-to-end anastomosis may be preferable, using the GIA instrument. A stab wound is made into the lumen of the proximal gastric tube to accommodate the anvil of the GIA instrument, and the cartridge fork is placed into the esophagus. The instrument halves are joined, the tissues evenly aligned, and the instrument closed and activated.

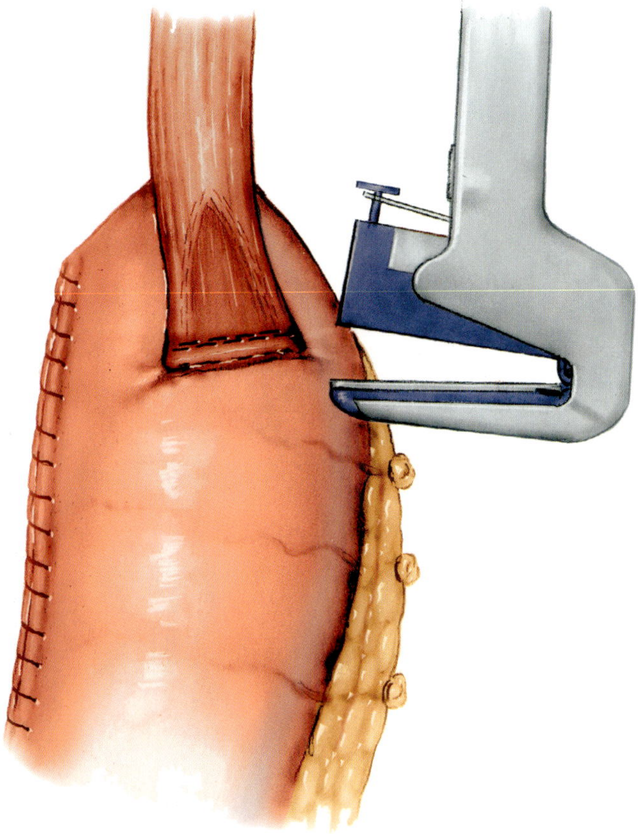

Figure III-6,H: Following removal of the instrument, the anastomosis is checked to ensure hemostasis prior to closure of the common opening. The staple lines at the open end of the anastomosis are held in opposition and the opening is closed transversely with a linear stapler, ensuring that all tissue layers and the ends of the GIA staple lines are incorporated in the closure.

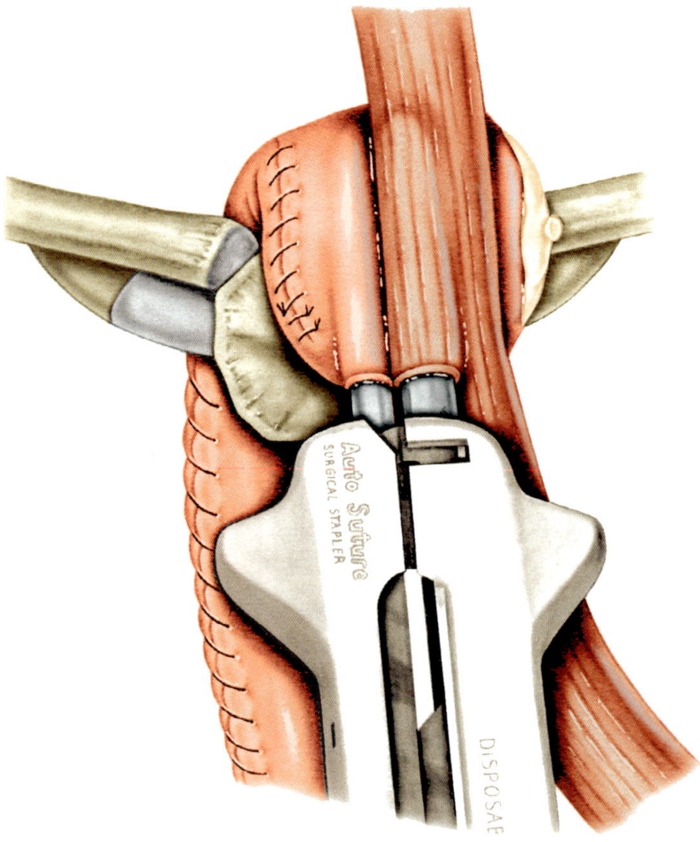

Figure III-6,I: The functional end-to-end anastomosis is facilitated by the use of the anastomosis first - resection second ("anastomose-resection integree") mode. Parallel stab wounds are made into the gastric tube and the esophagus at the site for the anastomosis. One fork of the GIA instrument is inserted into each lumen, and the instrument is closed and activated.

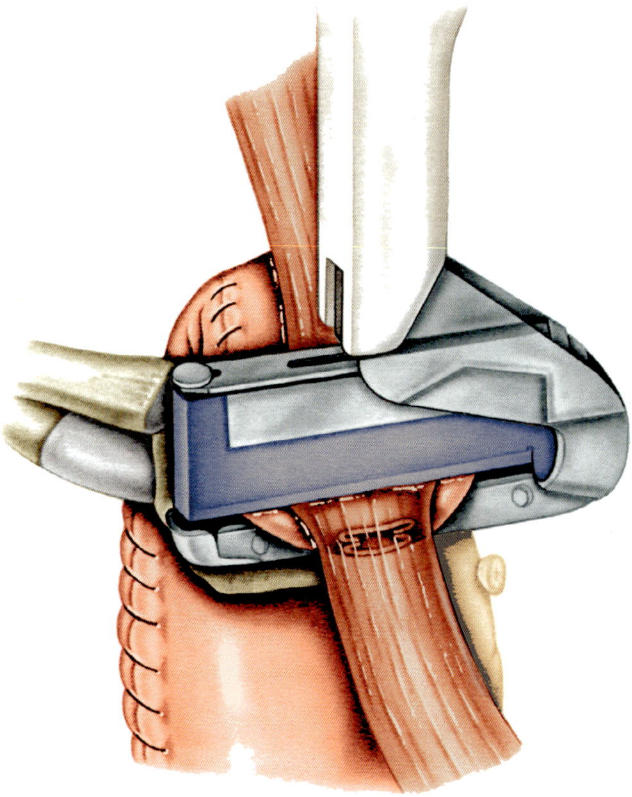

Figure III-6,J: Following accomplishment of the linear anastomosis and removal of the GIA instrument, the gastrotomy and esophagotomy, as well as the circumference of the esophagus, are closed with one application of the linear stapler, and the specimen is resected.

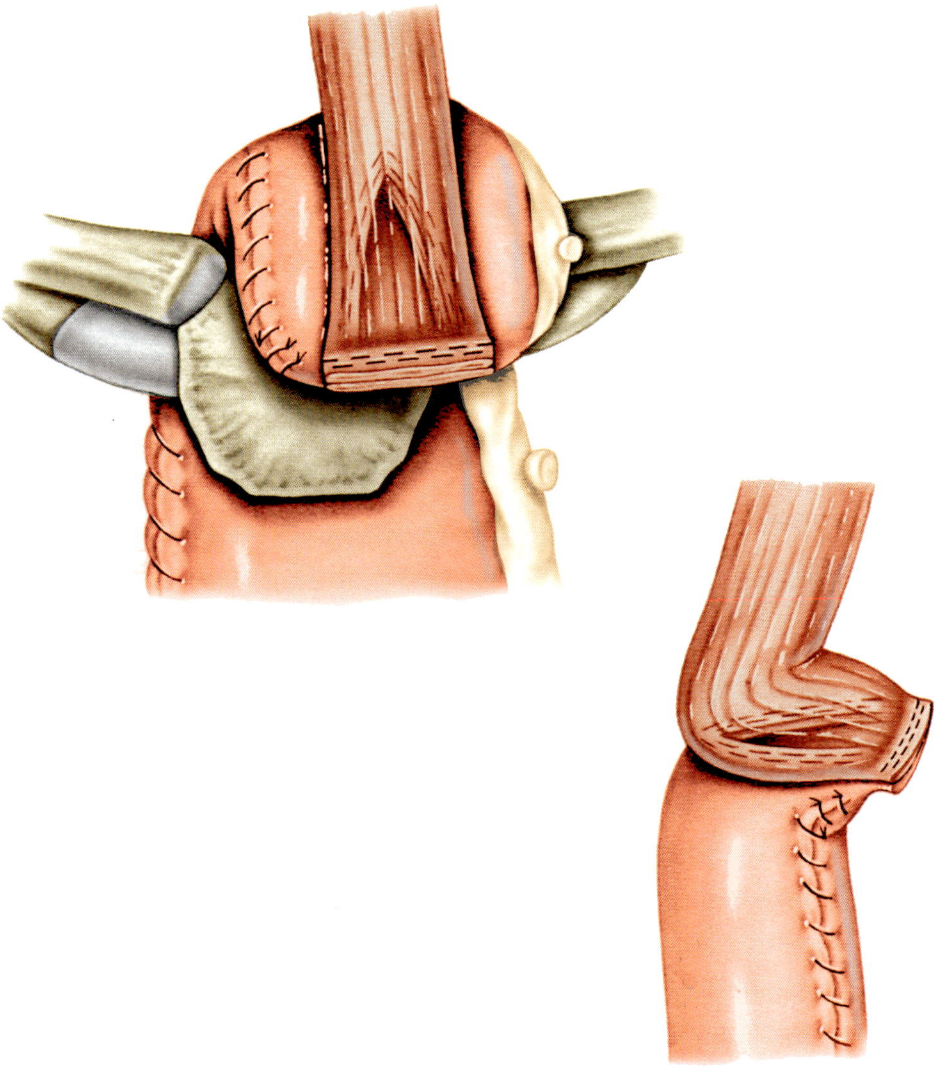

Figure III-6,K,L: The transverse linear staple line closes the common esophageal and gastric introduction sites, as well as the lumen of the esophagus. The final appearance of this closure is the same in both techniques: after resection of the esophagus first (Figure III-6, G and H) or resection second, following anastomosis done first (Figure III-6, I and J). A gentle pull on the stomach below the diaphragm straightens the functional end-to-end anastomosis into a tubular structure behind the clavicle.

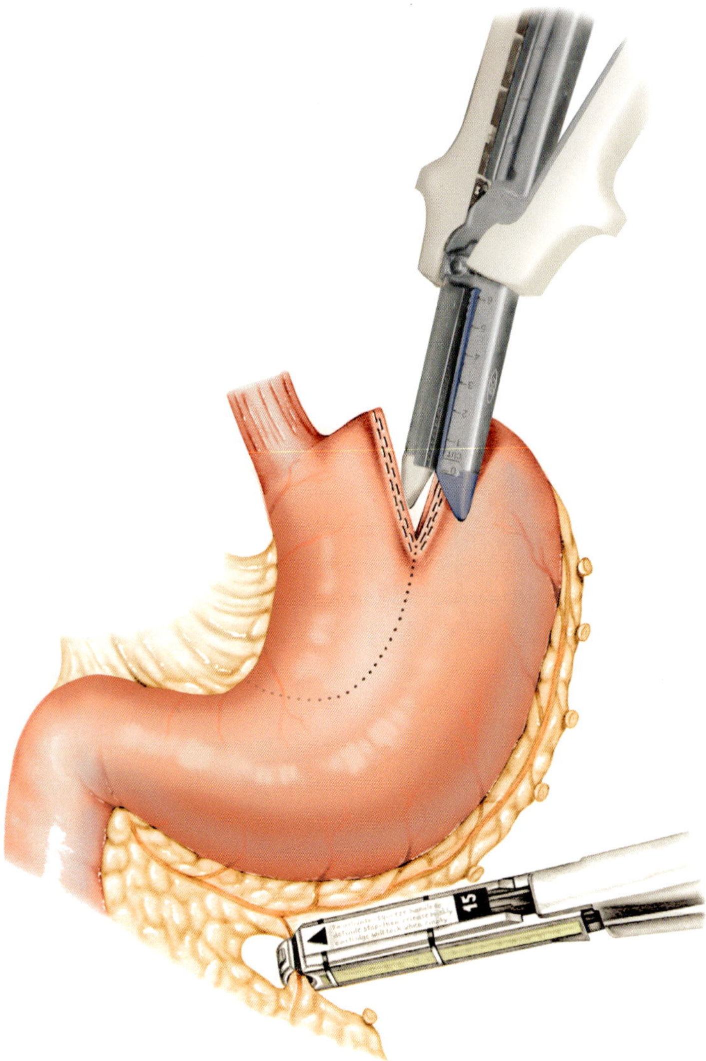

Figure III-6,M: In patients with lesions of the lower to middle third of the esophagus, where a left thoracoabdominal or separate left thoracic and abdominal approach have been used, proximal submucosal extension of the tumor may require a more cranial dissection, behind the arch of the aorta. In these cases, the remaining esophageal stump in the apex of the left chest has to be transposed in front of the arch of the aorta for anastomosis. In general, we try to avoid this technically more difficult solution by planning in such cases, if at all foreseeable, a right thoracic and separate midline abdominal approach for the dissection and substitute organ creation. This facilitates the anastomosis in the left or even right side of the neck or, alternatively, the apex of the right chest. If a left thoracoabdominal or separate left thoracic and abdominal approach have been used, following mobilization, the isoperistaltic tube may be fashioned from below (Figure III-6,A) or from above downward, using serial applications of the GIA instrument.

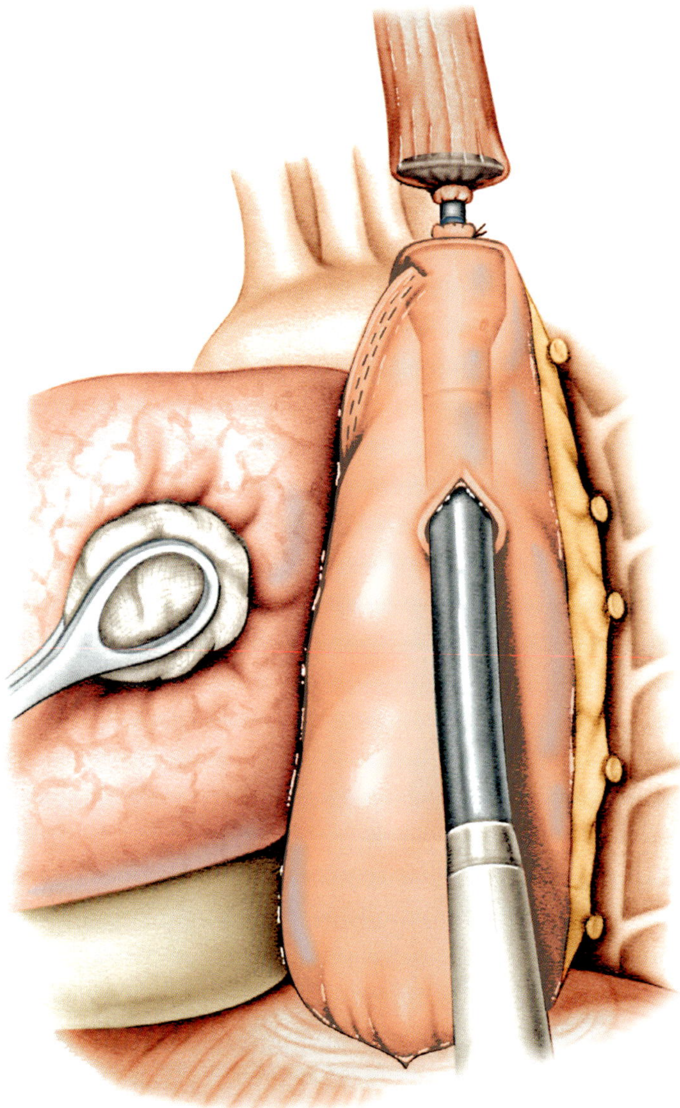

Figure III-6,N: The end-to-end circular anastomosis is performed with the EEA instrument placed through an anterior gastrotomy and the anvil placed separately into the esophagus as in Figure III-6,C. The gastrotomy is closed after removal of the EEA instrument as shown in Figure III-6,D.

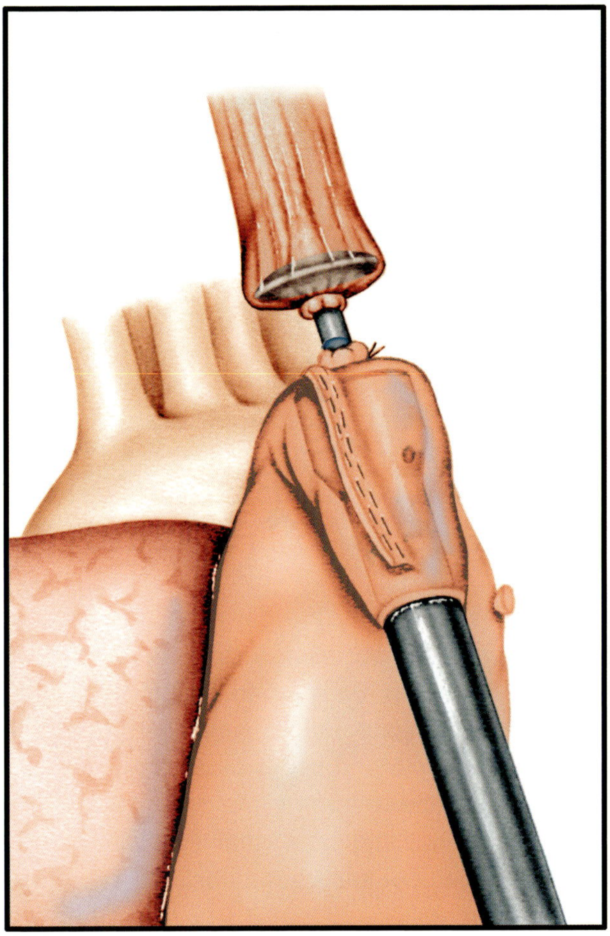

Figure III-6,O: If sufficient gastric tube is available and the blood supply to the tip of the tube is questionable, then an end-to-side anastomosis may be accomplished and the excess stomach excised peripheral to the circular anastomosis and linear closure with the TA instrument. As previously discussed, the gastric tube staple closure should be oversewn.

ESOPHAGOGASTRECTOMY AND ISOPERISTALTIC TUBE IN CONTINUITY WITH THE GASTRIC ANTRUM

This mode of replacement is best suited for the palliation of inoperable cancer of the thoracic esophagus, in patients whose general condition justifies this major operative approach. This esophageal substitute facilitates nutrition if and when radiotherapy is given. The reverse gastric tube (Figure III-3, A to K) and the elongated, tubular stomach (Figure III-6, A to O) may also be used as a bypass for inoperable middle and upper thoracic esophageal cancers. However, the isoperistaltic tube in continuity with the antrum is preferable since it maintains the original GE junction and drainage of the esophagus into the stomach below the tumor. It also allows passage of saliva and food along the parallel, but separate, substitute esophagus into the antrum of the remaining stomach.

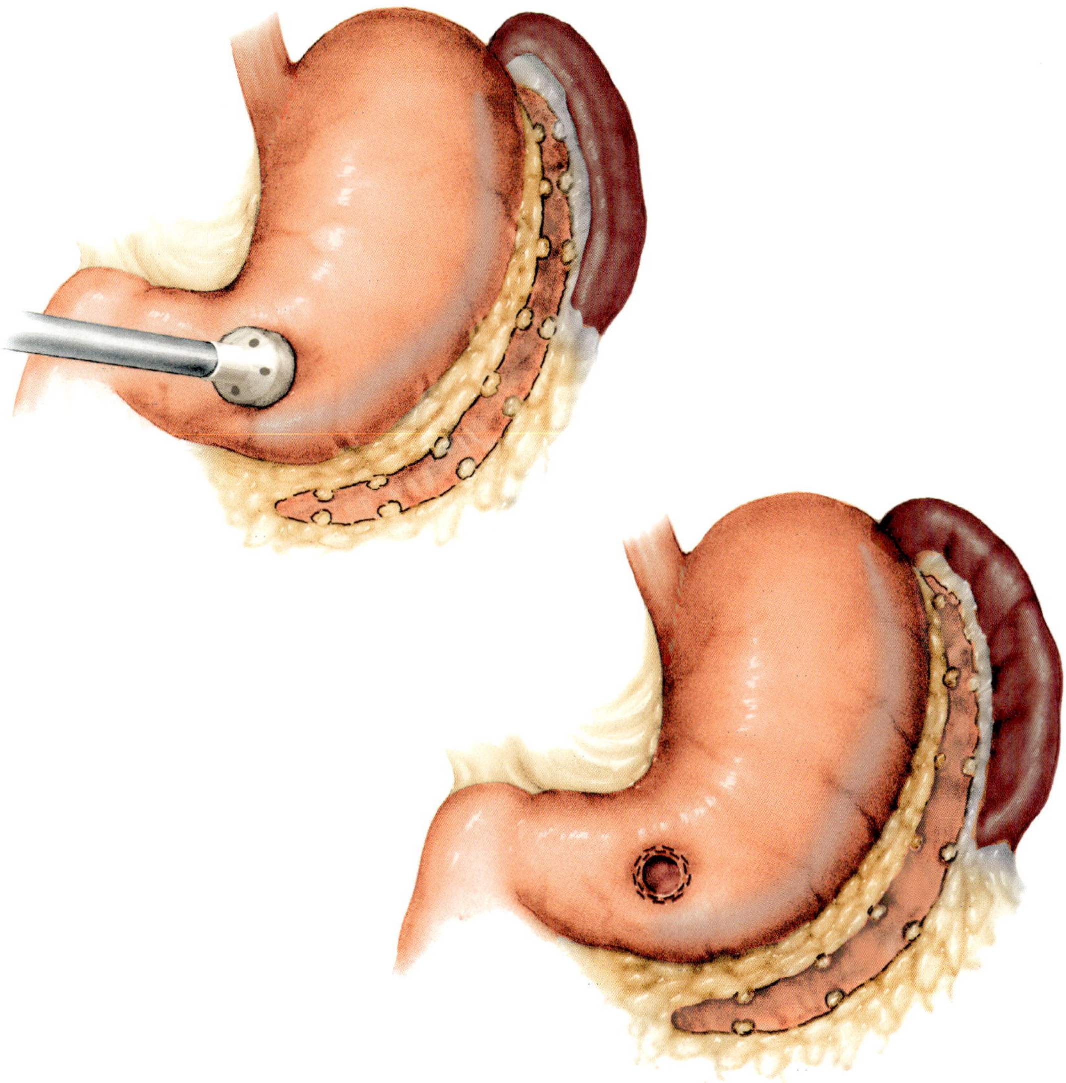

Figure III-7,A,B: The greater curvature of the stomach is mobilized, preserving the gastroepiploic vessels and the spleen. A buttonhole is created in the antrum, 3 to 4 cm proximal to the pylorus, closer to the greater than lesser curvature, with the EEA 21 instrument. The proposed tube is based on the right gastroepiploic artery and arcade.

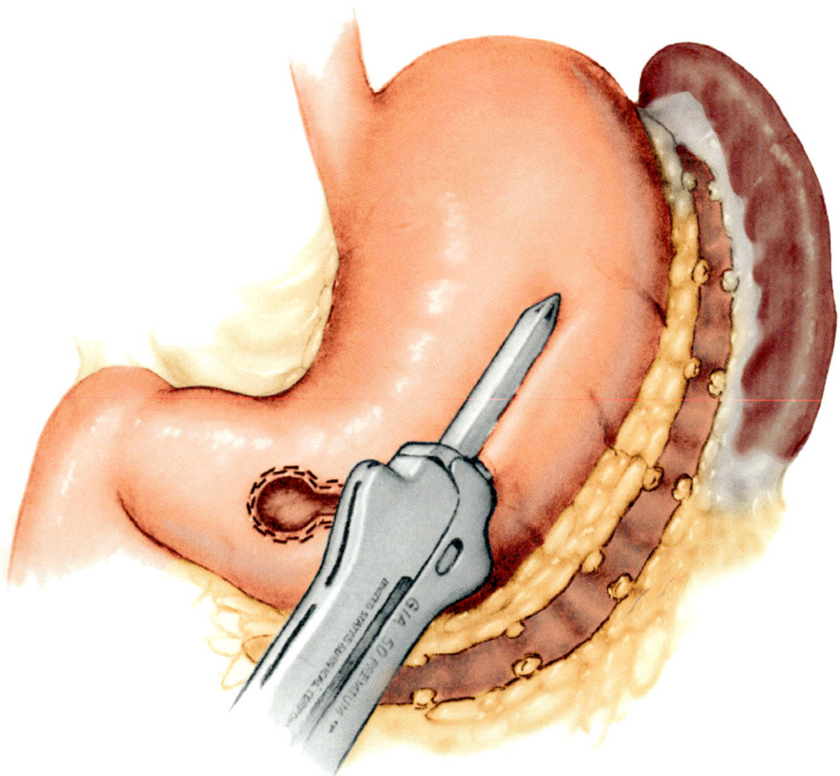

Figure III-7,C: One fork of the GIA instrument is placed through the antral buttonhole into the lesser sac, against the posterior wall, and the other fork is placed on the anterior wall of the stomach, inside and parallel to the greater curvature. As the instrument is closed and activated for the first time, it staples and cuts through the annular staple lines and outlines the shape of the future tube. The gastric tube is accomplished by serial applications of the GIA stapler in the direction of and beyond the apex of the fundus. With this technique, the spleen is always preserved, which makes it a favorite mode of esophageal replacement in children.

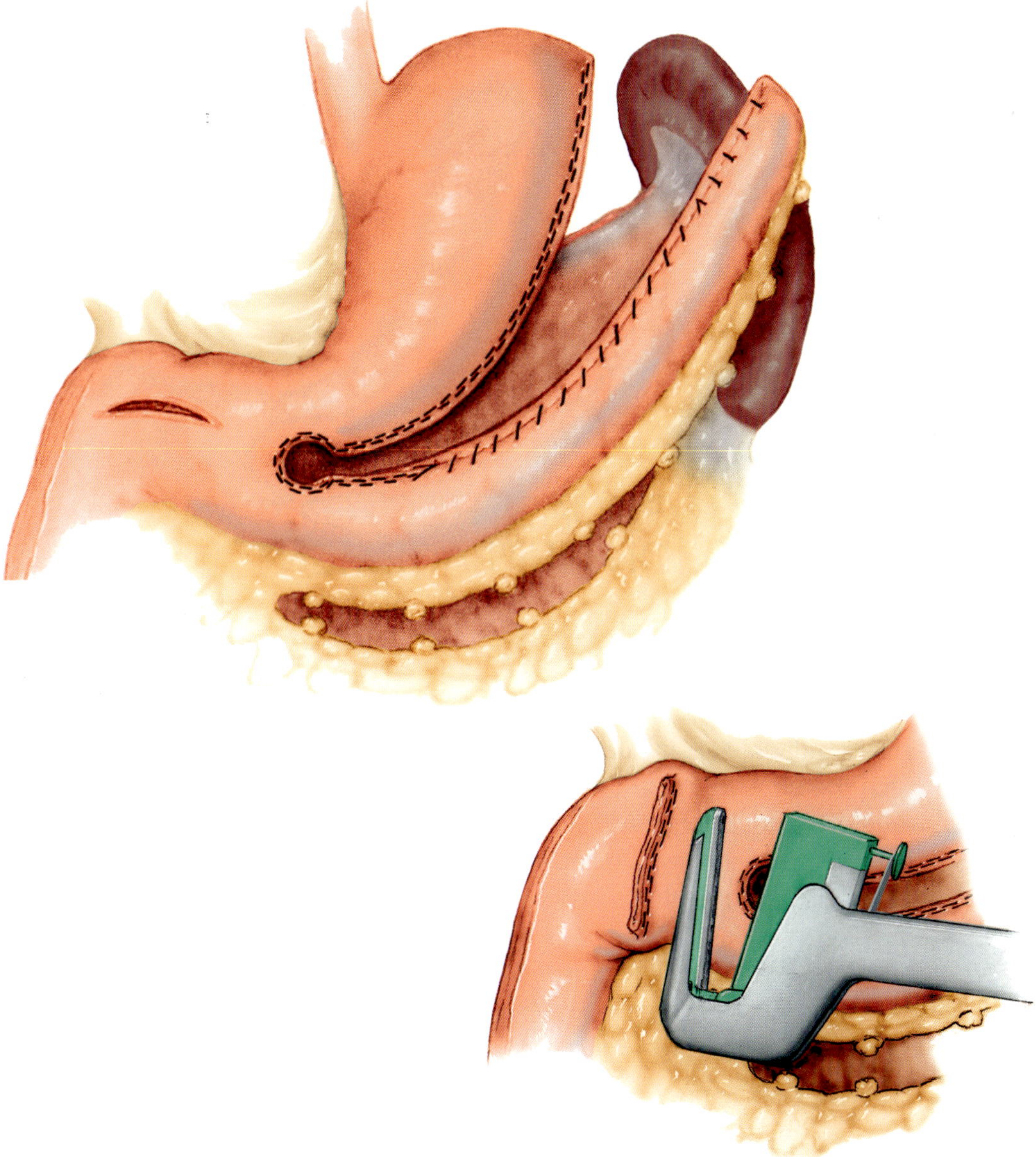

Figure III-7,D,E: As with other gastric tubes, the staple lines are oversewn, taking care to use interrupted sutures near the upper end of the tube, which is elevated into the neck through a retrosternal, anterior mediastinal channel. A Kocher maneuver is performed for added mobility to reach the desired height for the esophagogastrostomy. A Heineke-Mikulicz pyloroplasty is performed using a linear stapler.

ESOPHAGOGASTRECTOMY AND COLON REPLACEMENT

It has become obvious that no single method of substitute organ creation can satisfy the great variety of reconstructive features necessary to replace a given organ at all times, especially a structure like the esophagus that bridges three anatomical sites—the neck, the chest, and the abdomen. Therefore, if the entire stomach is not available, especially for esophageal substitutions that have to reach the neck or the apex of the chest, the right or left colon represents a good alternative. This is also true in children, in whom a long reverse gastric tube might result in a planned or "incidental" splenectomy. Although we have a good experience in replacing the lower esophagus and the GE junction with a segment of jejunum, we have avoided the use of the small bowel in higher locations because of obvious technical difficulties related to the shortness of the mesentery and the anatomically limited span of the blood supply.

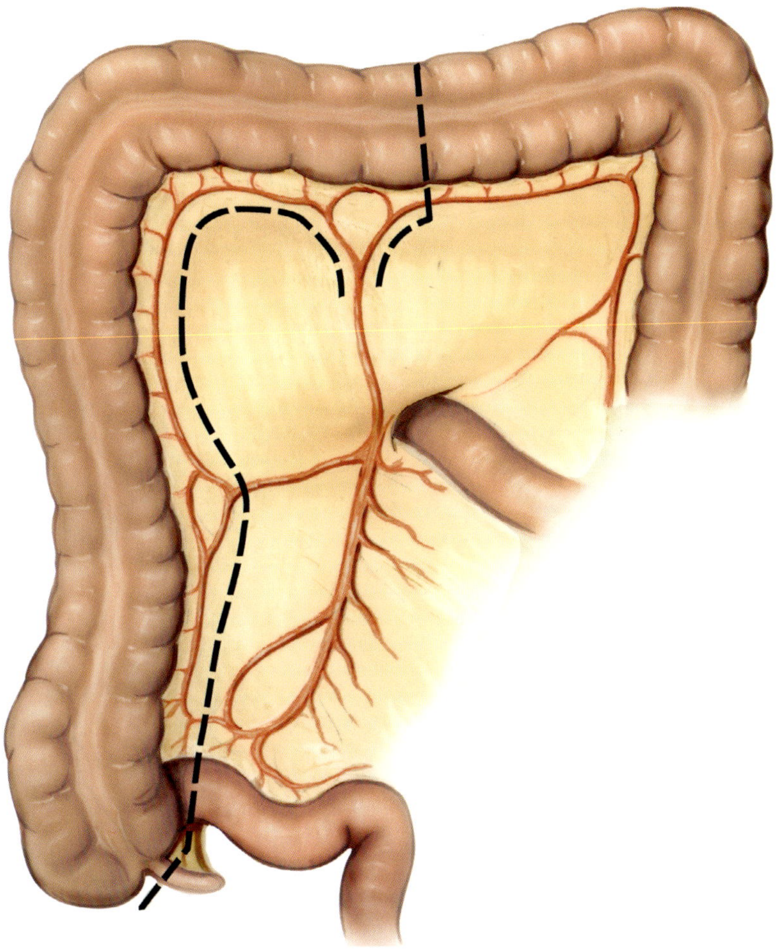

Figure III-8,A: The selection of a suitable segment of colon for esophageal replacement varies depending on the extent of esophageal resection, the vascularity and mobility of the colon segment, and the surgeon's preference. In the case of the right colon (illustrated in the following procedure), the ileocecal, right colic, and left branch of the middle colic vessels are ligated and divided to provide the viable, mobile segment.

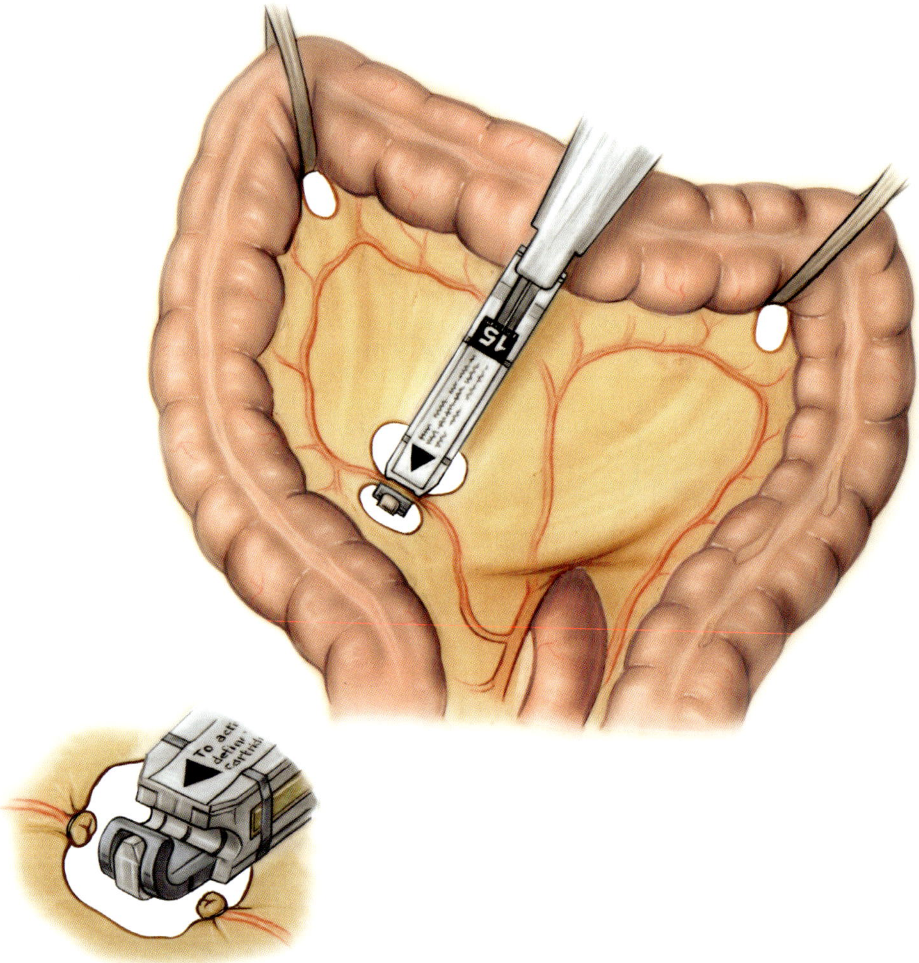

Figure III-8,B,C: Ligation and division of the vessels and subsequent mobilization of the colon can be expedited with the use of the LDS instrument, which places two crescent-shaped staples and simultaneously cuts evenly between them.

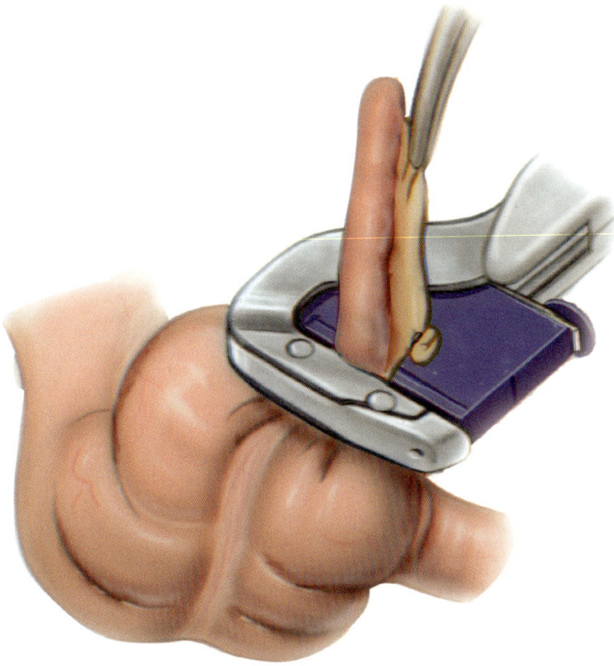

Figure III-8,D: The appendiceal vessels have been secured, and the appendix is amputated using the TA 30 (as shown) or GIA instrument.

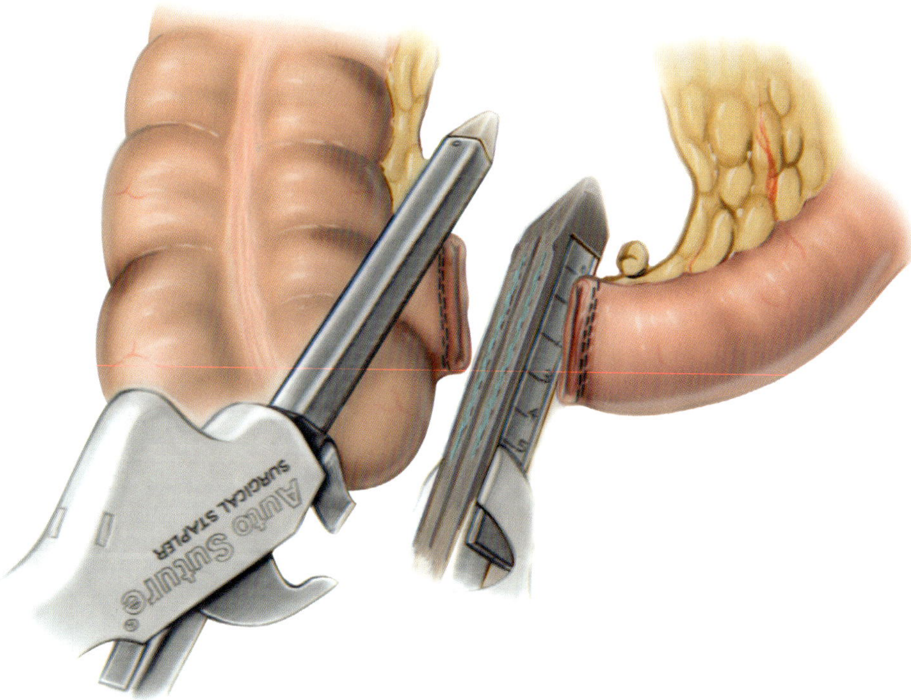

Figure III-8,E: The terminal ileum is closed on each side of the transection with the GIA instrument just proximal to the ileocecal valve.

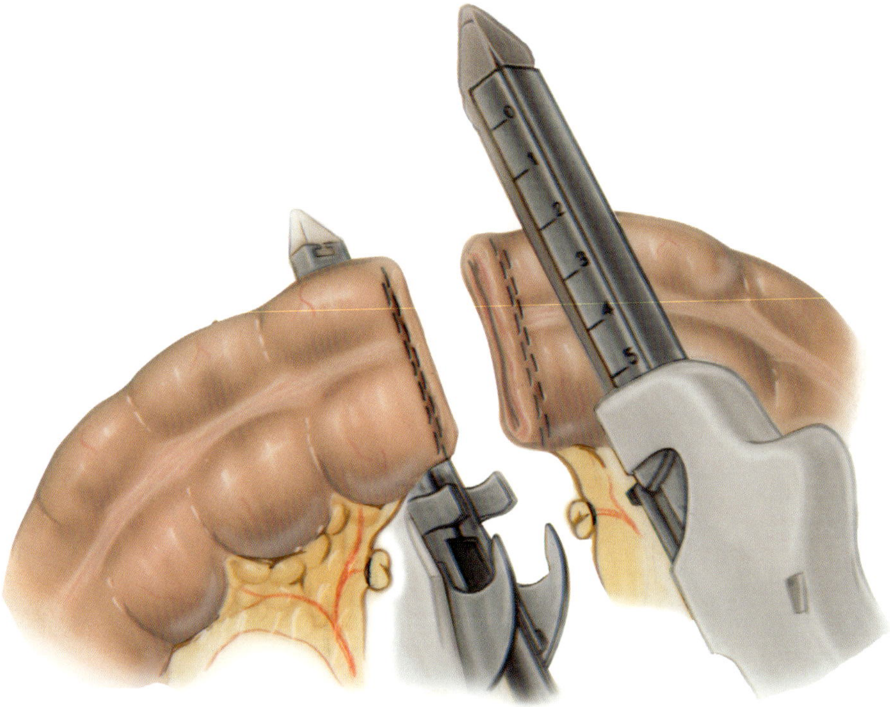

Figure III-8,F: The transverse colon is similarly stapled and divided to the left of the middle colic vessels with the GIA instrument.

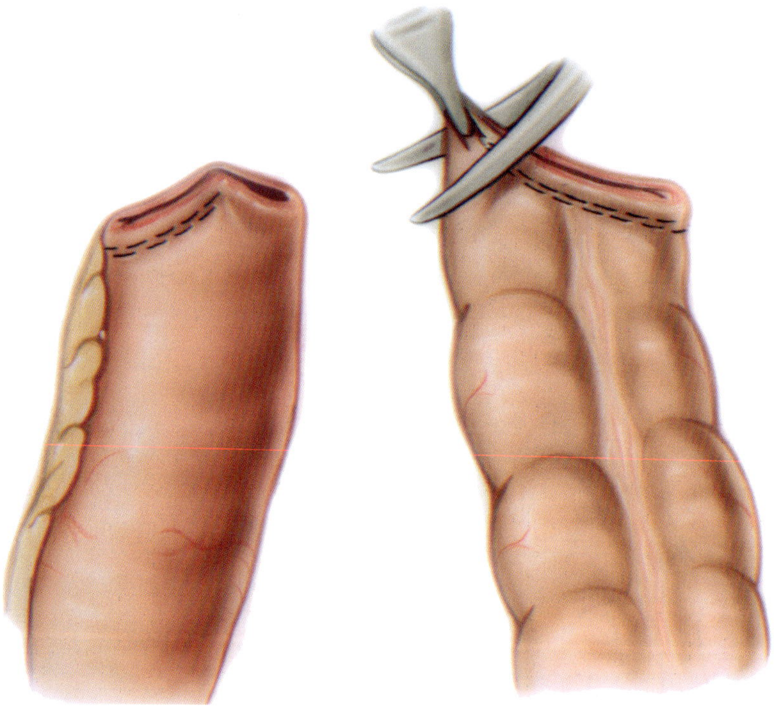

Figure III-8,G: An ileo-transverse colostomy is performed, using the functional end-to-end anastomotic technique, to restore intestinal continuity. The antimesenteric corners of the closed ileum and transverse colon are excised.

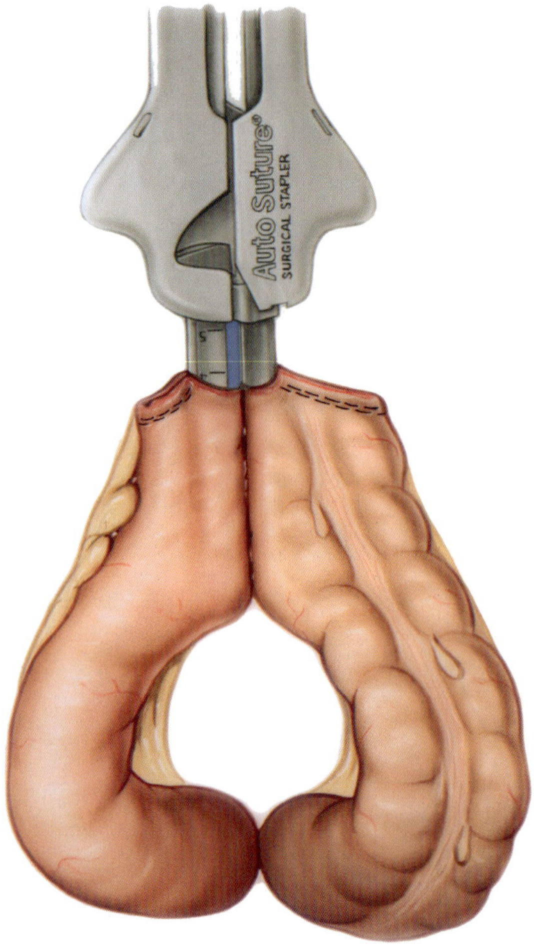

Figure III-8,H: One fork of the GIA instrument is inserted into each lumen. The instrument halves are joined and the bowel ends are evenly aligned on the forks of the instrument. The instrument is closed, compressing the antimesenteric bowel walls, and the instrument is activated, creating a side-to-side anastomosis. Following removal of the instrument, the anastomosis is checked to ensure hemostasis.

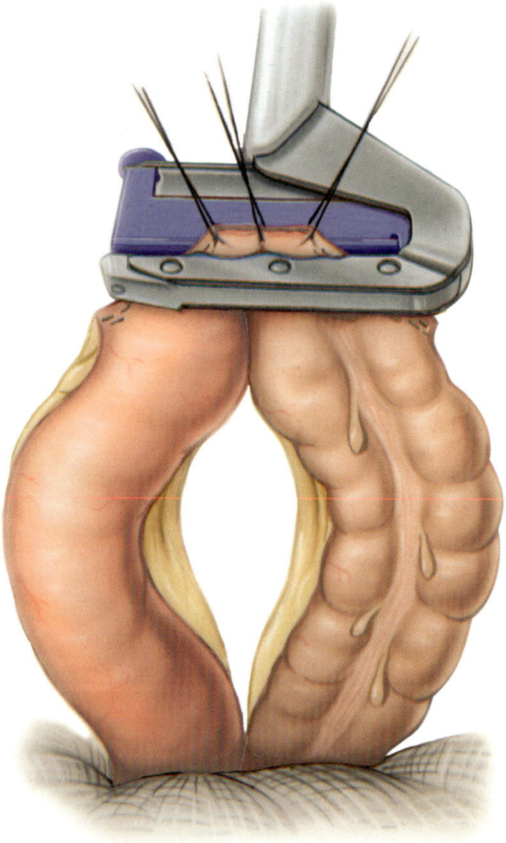

Figure III-8,I: The now common opening is closed with a linear stapler, taking care to include the entire circumference of the opening, all tissue layers, and the ends of all staple lines. When closing the instrument, the anastomotic staple lines should be juxtaposed to avoid their superposition. Following activation of the instrument, the excess tissue is excised along the instrument edge prior to removing the stapler. An anchor suture may be placed at the distal end of the anastomosis for additional security. Although anatomically a side-to-side anastomosis, postoperatively, this mode of joining two bowel ends will function as an end-to-end anastomosis.

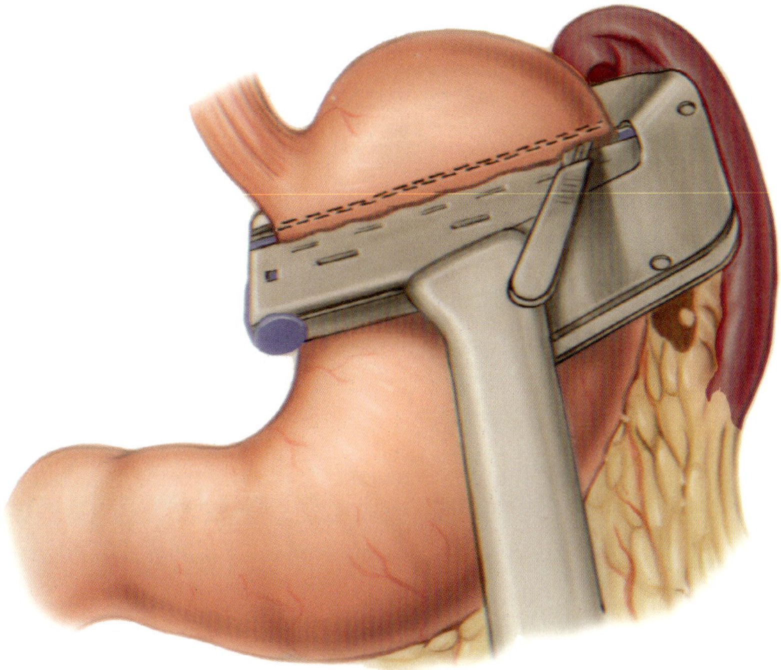

Figure III-8,J: The gastric fundus is amputated, in this instance between two applications of the TA 90 instrument. Following the first application, the TA 90 instrument is reapplied parallel and distal to the first staple line. Prior to removing the instrument, the stomach is transected between the two double staple lines along the superior edge of the stapler.

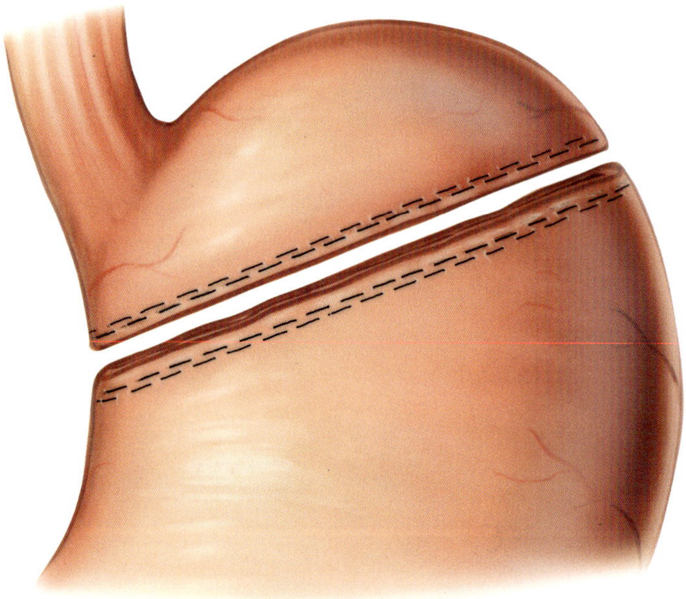

Figure III-8,K: Closure of both the remaining gastric pouch and specimen reduces the potential for intraperitoneal contamination.

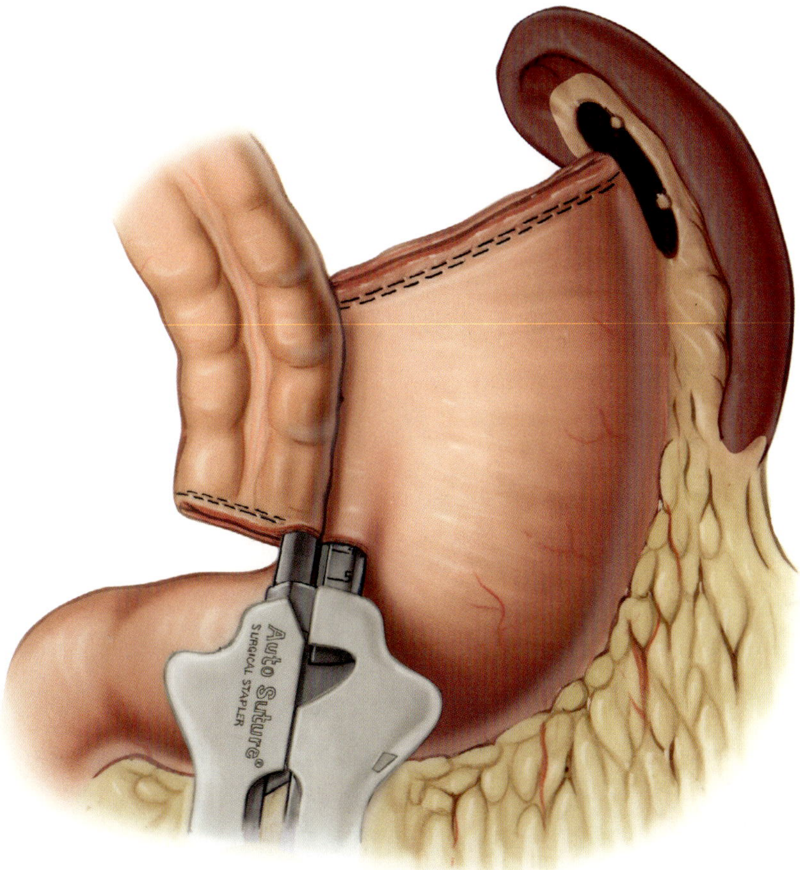

Figure III-8,L: The colon and its vascular pedicle are brought up behind the stomach into the anterior or posterior mediastinum, and the terminolateral anastomosis is performed between the colon and the stomach. The forks of the GIA instrument are inserted through the excised antimesenteric corner of the colon staple line and a stab wound in the remaining mid-lesser curvature of the stomach. The instrument halves are mated, and the instrument is closed and activated.

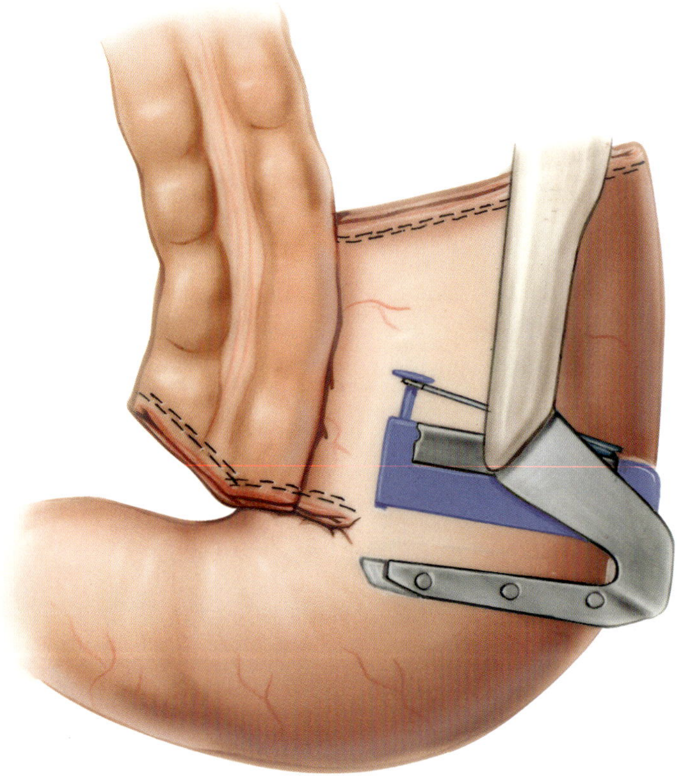

Figure III-8,M: Following removal of the GIA instrument, the cologastrostomy is inspected for hemostasis. The resultant single opening is closed mucosa-to-mucosa with the TA instrument, once again taking care to include the entire circumference of the opening, all tissue layers, and the ends of all staple lines.

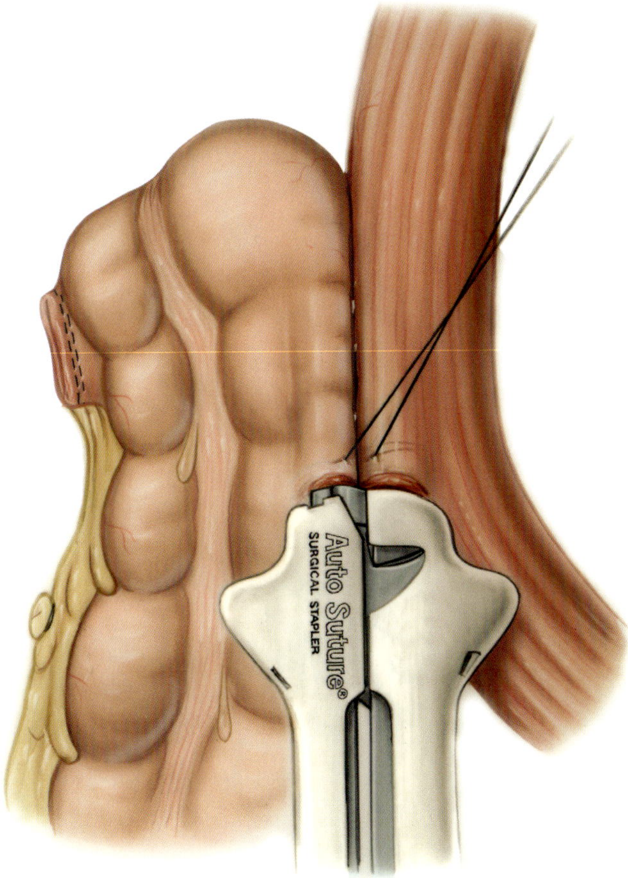

Figure III-8,N: The cecum is elevated into the neck, placed alongside the cervical esophagus, and the GIA instrument is passed cephalad through stab wounds in the antimesenteric border of the cecum and the lateral wall of the esophagus. The instrument is closed and activated.

While the approach to the cervical esophagus is somewhat easier through a left cervical incision, it can be performed through a right-sided cervicotomy if the overall positioning of the patient on the table requires this. Similarly, the esophagocolostomy can therefore be placed on the right or left lateral aspect of the esophagus.

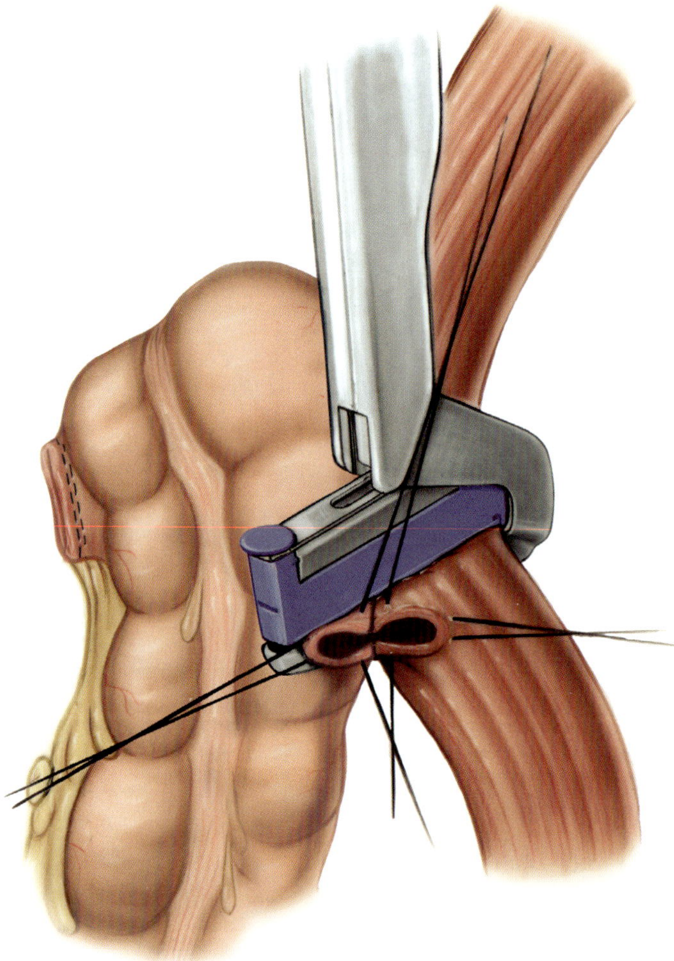

Figure III-8,O: With the GIA instrument withdrawn and after the anastomosis has been inspected, the appropriate placement of the TA instrument allows the esophagus to be stapled off obliquely, including the now common GIA instrument opening, so that when the esophagus is cut away with the scalpel along the inferior edge of the instrument, the resulting anastomosis in effect is end-to-end. This overlapping or bayonet-type reconstruction is applicable also to low rectal anastomoses ("anastomose-resection integree").

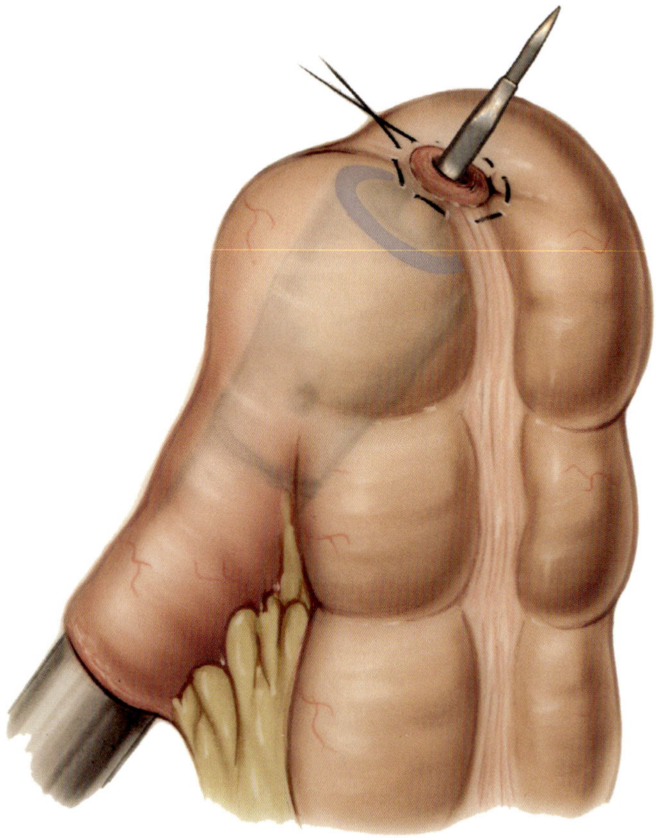

Figure III-8,P: Alternatively, the esophagocolostomy may be performed using the EEA instrument placed through the lumen of the distal ileum. The cartridge is advanced to the site for anastomosis and the instrument is opened, allowing the center rod to perforate the antimesocolic border of the cecum, which is then secured with a manual purse-string suture around the center rod.

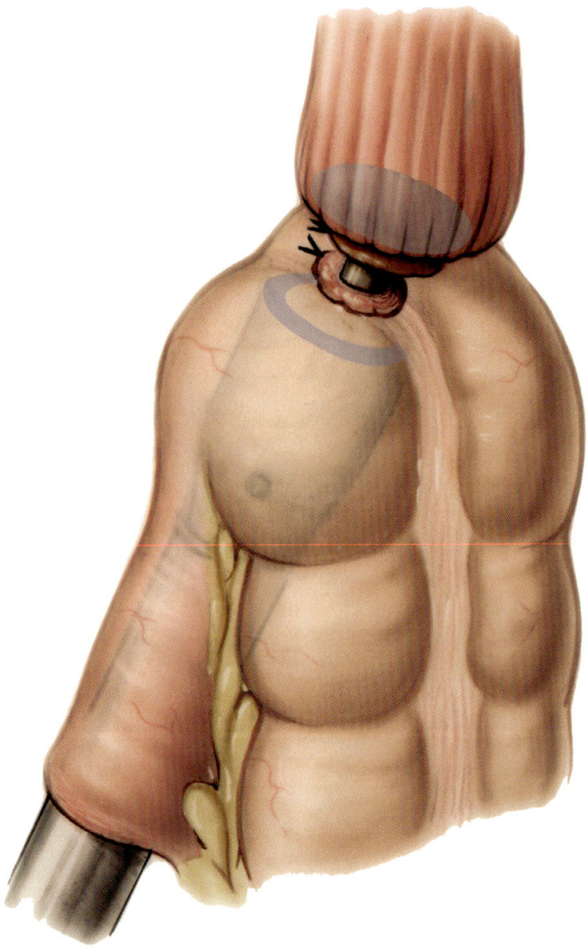

Figure III-8,Q: The proximal esophagus is prepared with a purse-string suture. The anvil is positioned in the esophagus, and the suture is tied securely on the anvil shaft. Ensuring that the tissue is snug against the cartridge and anvil reduces the possibility of any bunching or overlapping of tissue as the instrument is closed. The anvil shaft and center rod are joined, and the instrument is closed and activated. The instrument places a circular, double staggered row of staples and cuts the esophagocolic stoma.

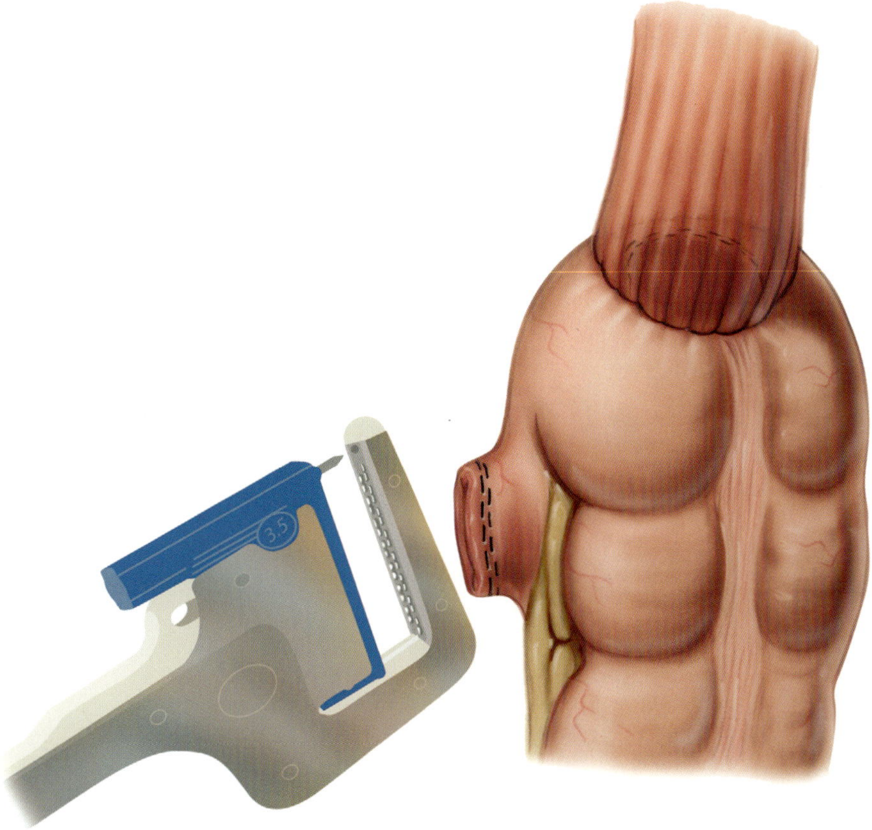

Figure III-8,R: Following removal of the EEA instrument, the anastomosis is inspected for hemostasis and the excised tissue “donuts” remaining in the instrument are checked to ensure that all tissue layers and purse-string sutures are intact. The distal ileum is closed with a linear stapling instrument.

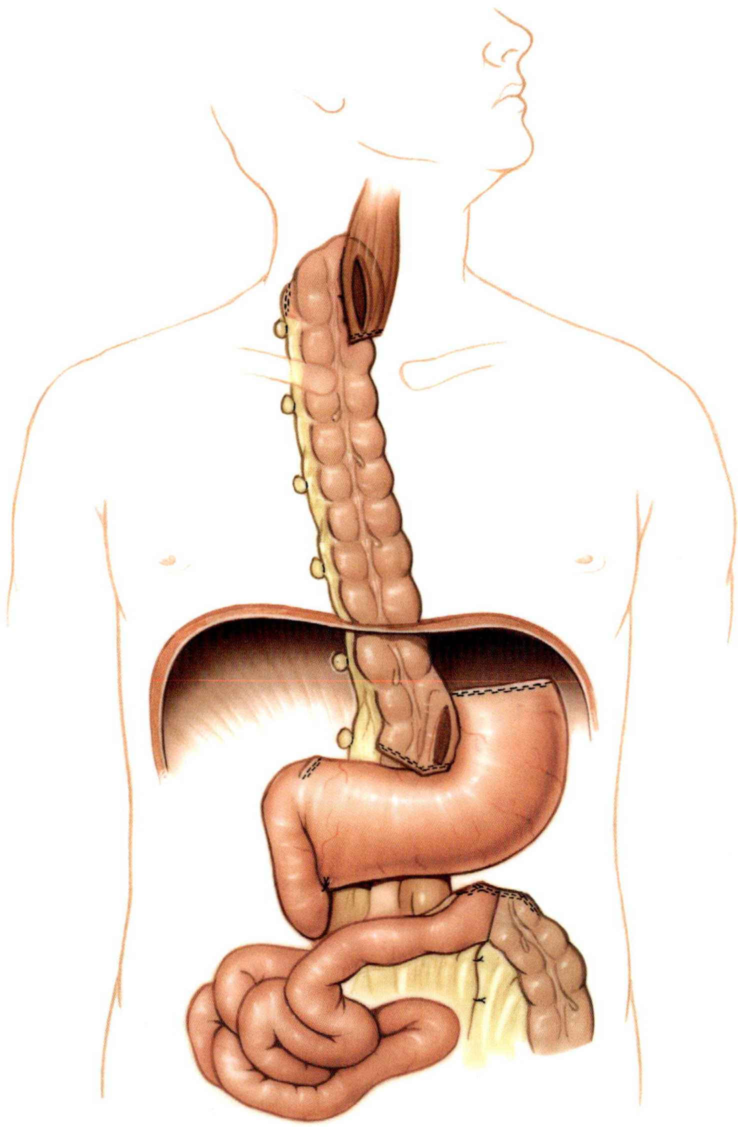

Figure III-8,S: The completed reconstruction showing the closure and transection of the ileum, transverse colon, and gastric fundus, appendectomy, Finney pyloroplasty, functional end-to-end ileocolostomy, end-to-side cologastrostomy, and end-to-side esophagocolostomy involves 14 staple lines. In general, we find that the great merit of the instruments lies in their precision and neatness, in the decrease in the trauma inflicted on the tissues, and in the lessened opportunity for bleeding or contamination. In operations as extensive as that shown, the time saved to the patient also becomes a major factor.

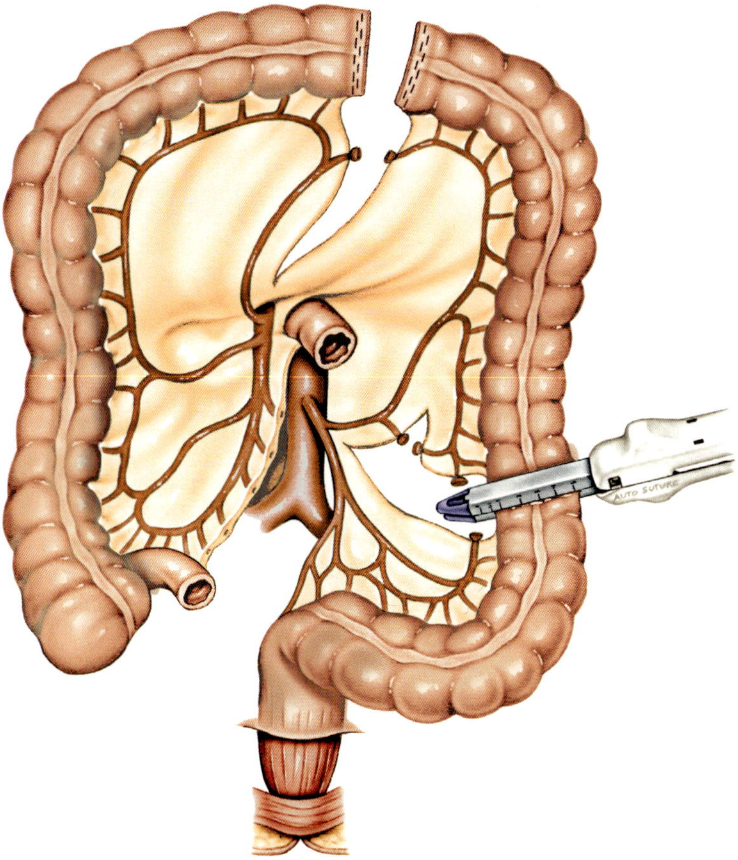

Figure III-8,T: If a left colon segment is preferred for replacement, the left branches of the middle colic vessels and the descending branches of the left colic vessels will be ligated and divided; the colon segment is based on the vessels ascending from the left colic artery and vein. If possible, this segment should be used in an isoperistaltic fashion. In fact, it is most often composed of the distal transverse colon, the splenic flexure, and the descending colon, based on the ascending branch of the left colic artery (itself a branch of the inferior mesenteric artery) and the corresponding marginal artery of Drummond. The descending left colic branch may limit mobility of the colon segment and will then require careful ligation and transection between its origin from the left colic artery and its junction with the marginal artery. The transection between the descending and sigmoid colon is pursued medially in the avascular mesocolon, between the left colic and sigmoid arteries, after ligation and transection of the marginal vessels. At times, adequate mobility of the left transverse and descending colon segment appears easier if it is based on the left branch of the middle colic artery and elevated into the neck in an antiperistaltic fashion. Although the colon is usually considered to be an atonic conduit, reverse peristalsis has been observed with this mode of replacement.

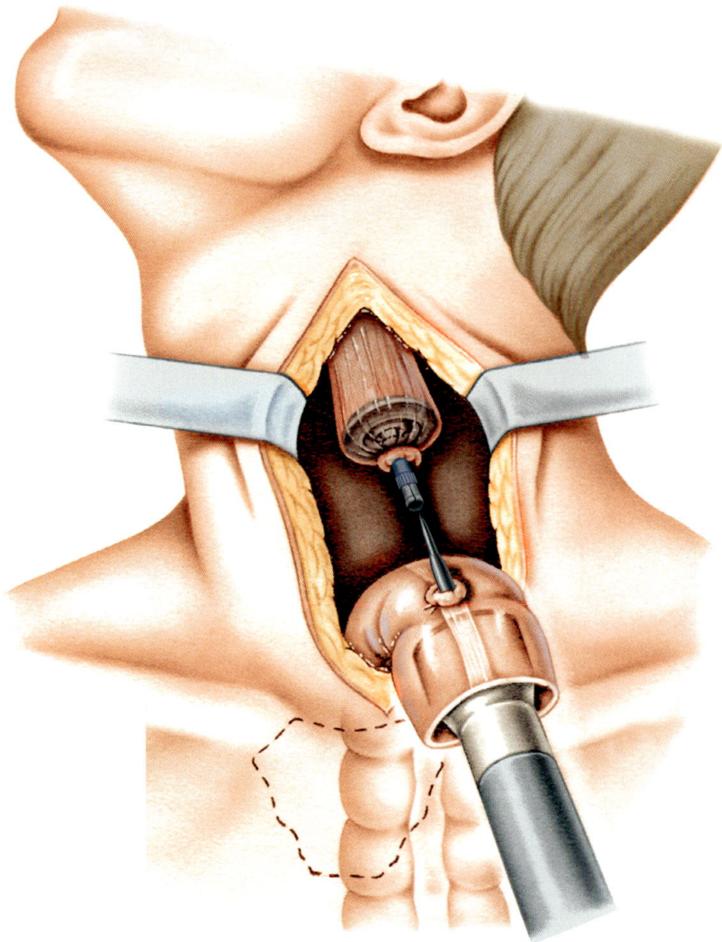

Figure III-8,U: If use of the left colon presents an open lumen in the neck, esophagocolostomy may be performed manually, with a posterior and anterior running suture, incorporating all layers of both ends. The anastomosis may also be accomplished with interrupted sutures as shown in Figure III-3,I for the reverse gastric tube. We, as well as others, have found no advantage or greater safety with a layered anastomosis, and we use additional sutures only to reinforce here and there.

If the colon segment is of sufficient length, mechanical circular anastomosis is possible by flexing the excess colon like a cane. The anvil is separately secured in the cervical esophagus with a purse-string suture. The EEA instrument with cartridge is placed into the lumen of the curved colon, the instrument's center rod is advanced through the antimesocolic wall at the apex of the curve, and the tissue is secured with a manual purse-string suture. The anvil shaft and center rod are joined, and the instrument is closed and activated.

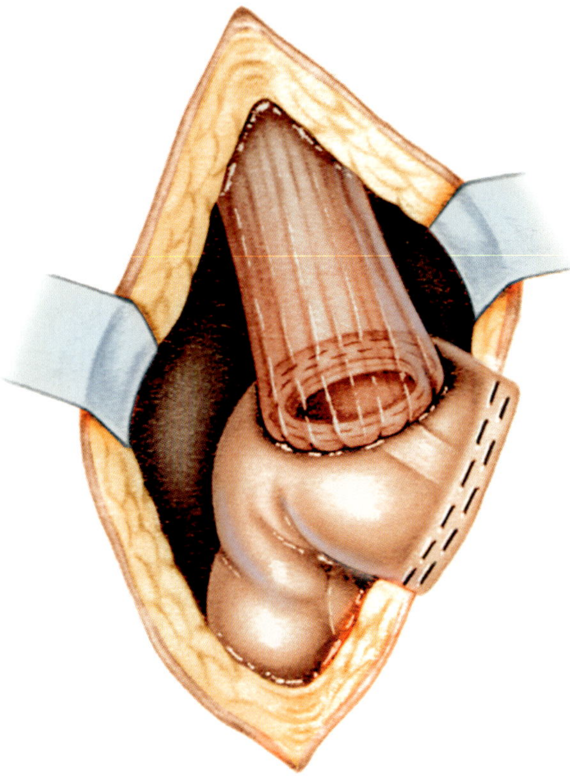

Figure III-8,V: Following satisfactory anastomosis, disengagement of the circular stapling instrument, and inspection, the remaining colon cane stump is closed with a linear stapler and the excess colon excised.

An anterior pylorectomy can be performed with the EEA 25 instrument placed through the gastrotomy, which is used later for the cologastrostomy.

ESOPHAGOGASTRECTOMY AND COLON REPLACEMENT IN THE CHILD

As any possible compromise to the spleen must be avoided at all costs in children, we prefer replacing the esophagus with a segment of large bowel. While raising a reverse gastric tube in a child without removing the spleen is technically possible and satisfies in most cases both function and distance, we prefer to steer clear of the vascular junction represented by the splenic and left gastroepiploic vessels. The segment most often chosen is the transverse colon—it is easy to mobilize in children, and it allows conservation of the ileocecal valve and of the more deeply attached descending colon. In most instances, it is of sufficient length to bridge almost any defect; if needed, extra length can be obtained by using part or all of the splenic flexure. Depending on the configuration and mobility of the mid-colic vessels and their branches, it can be used in an isoperistaltic mode based on the left mid-colic vessel branches or in an antiperistaltic fashion based on the right mid-colic vessel branches. Although the large bowel performs well as a substitute esophagus, it has a tendency to sag and form a buckle or siphon at the distal colon to esophageal stump or stomach anastomosis as the child grows into adulthood. Therefore, it is important to tailor the segment of colon to the exact length required to bridge the esophageal defect and to construct a distal anastomosis that will cause neither obstruction nor massive reflux, a difficult task. Despite taking these precautionary measures, these anastomoses have to be revised occasionally in adult age because of stasis and regurgitation from the colic siphon. In children, esophageal replacement may be necessary because of a long atresia after a failed primary reconstruction of a TE fistula or because of a long atresia without fistula. If a distal esophageal stump is available for anastomosis, which is most often the case, it should be carefully preserved and used in order to maintain a competent GE junction (the Waterston principle). If esophageal substitution is needed for replacement after a lye burn, the usual extent of substitution is from neck to abdomen.

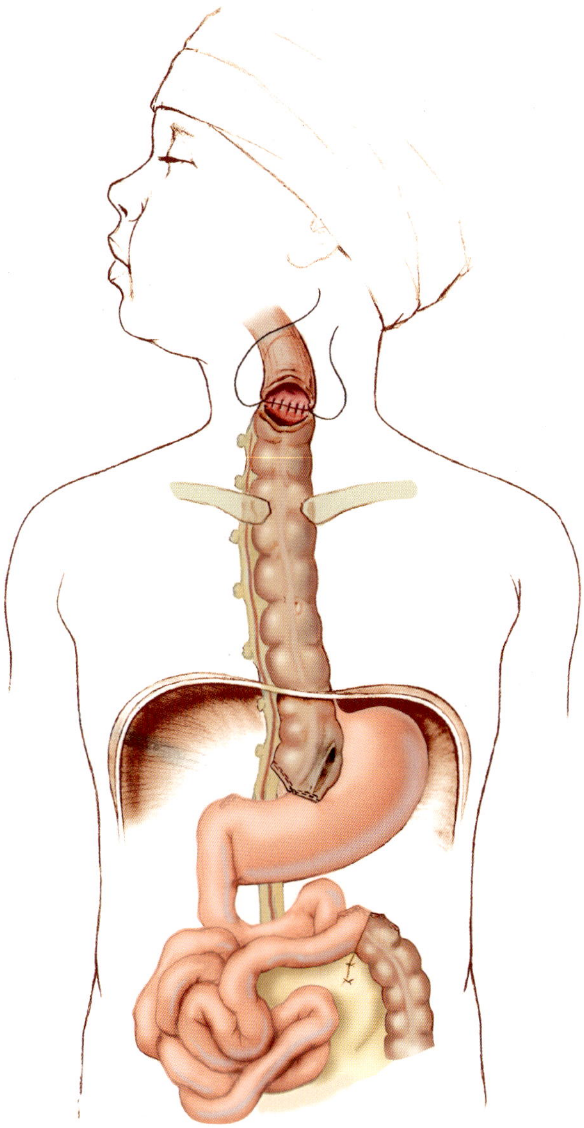

Figure III-9,A: A complete esophageal reconstruction for lye burn is shown. In this patient, the right colon was used to securely bridge a rather extensive defect. In the neck, the anastomosis to the cecum (or colon) is a manual one, since in children of this age even the smallest EEA and GIA instruments are too large and awkward to position. The articulated ENDO GIA stapler may be used to perform the anastomosis in the bigger child and the teenager, for whom this operation is, hopefully, rarely, if ever, necessary. In this patient, all bowel closures and remaining anastomoses were performed with mechanical sutures—closure and transection of the ileum and transverse colon, functional end-to-end ileocolostomy, Finney pyloroplasty, and end-to-side cologastrostomy.

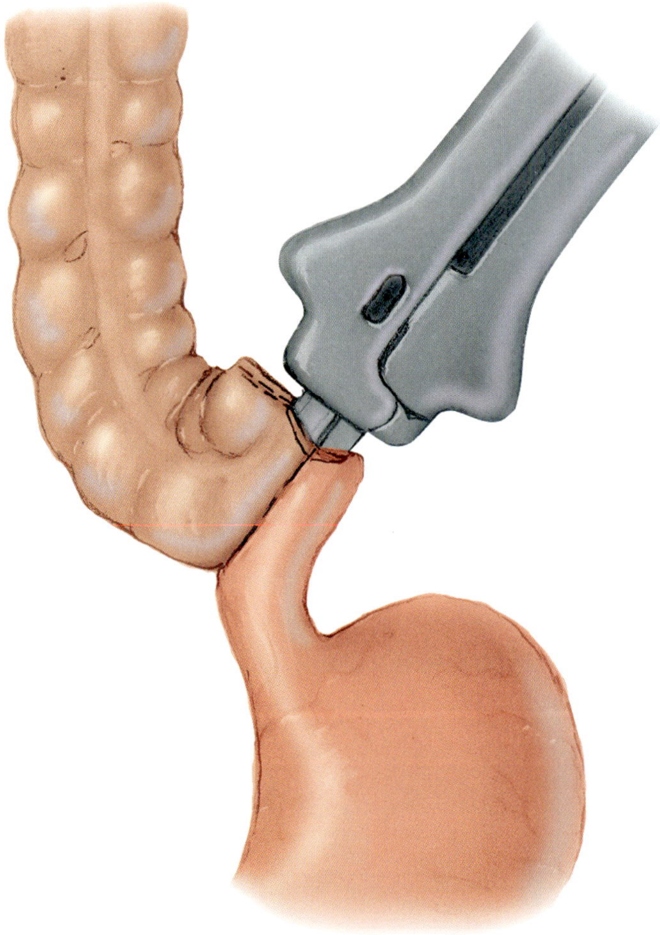

Figure III-9,B: The Waterston reconstruction can be performed in children with a wide-gap—primary or secondary—esophageal atresia. The colon segment is raised into the posterior mediastinum, and the distal esophageal stump is used for anastomosis to the distal end of the colon. The GIA instrument is used to create a functional end-to-end anastomosis.

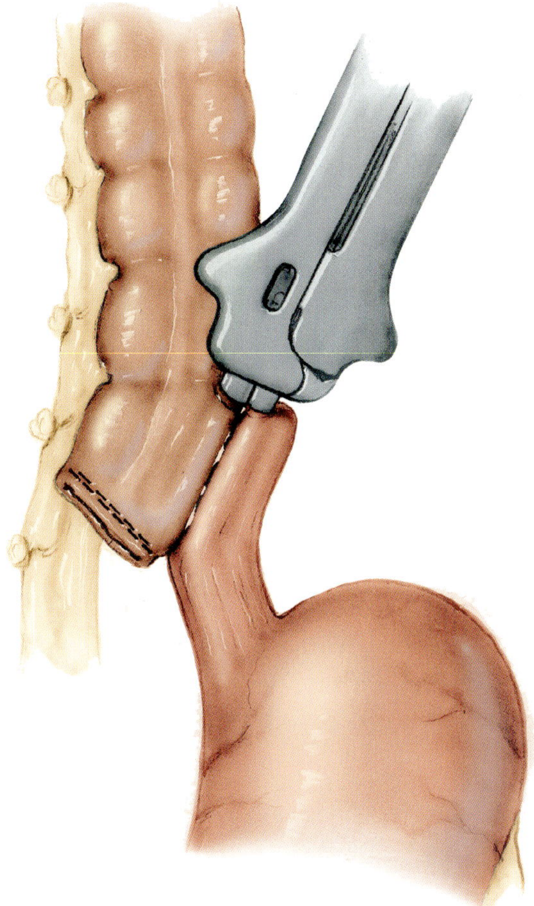

Figure III-9,C: Alternatively, the anastomosis can be performed in a bayonet mode. In either case, following removal of the GIA instrument and inspection of the anastomosis, the common opening is closed with a linear stapler.

Note: If circumstances in a given patient did not respect the integrity of the GE junction and gastroesophageal reflux represents a real threat to the coloesophageal anastomosis during the postoperative period and later, then an antireflux operation of the Toupet type is indicated. If the distal esophageal stump is short and does not allow a safe repositioning of the entire stomach below the diaphragm, a Collis-Toupet operation is indicated, similar to a Collis-Nissen operation in the adult. We do not favor a complete Nissen fundoplication in children with the colo-distal esophageal anastomosis described above, since the initial slow passage and stasis of air and saliva at the level of the fundoplication may compromise the coloesophageal anastomosis.

MECHANICAL SUTURES IN OPERATIONS ON THE LOWER ESOPHAGUS AND GASTROESOPHAGEAL JUNCTION BY THORACOTOMY AND LAPAROTOMY

The indications for radical surgery at this level are, in the majority of cases, the various forms of squamous cell cancer and adenocarcinoma. In cancers of the middle and upper third of the esophagus, lymph node dissection below the diaphragm, together with excision of the lesser curvature, is only required if the nodes contain metastatic deposits and/or the need exists to elongate the stomach into a tube. In contrast, cancers of the lower esophagus and gastric cardia always require lymph node dissection of the celiac axis and its distribution, as well as a tumor-dependent resection of the fundus and lesser curvature and possibly splenectomy. This leaves a shorter, broad or narrow gastric tube that can be anastomosed to the tumor-free (by intraoperative histological examination) mid-to-upper esophagus and that is based on the right gastroepiploic vessels.

Alternatively, if the gap between the esophagus and stomach is too wide, a segment of colon can be interposed. With either mode of esophageal substitution, the anastomosis to the esophagus can take place in the right or left chest through an appropriate thoracotomy or in the mediastinum through the diaphragmatic hiatus exposed by laparotomy, which is always required for the creation of the substitute organ and the celiac area lymphadenectomy. We prefer separate thoracotomy and laparotomy to the use of the combined left thoracoabdominal incision because of an increased incidence of wound-related postoperative complications with the latter type of incision. Besides the technical challenge of each individual dissection and excision, if indicated, the area of the distal esophagus and of the gastroesophageal junction require variety and flexibility of available reconstructive procedures in order to satisfy the therapeutic outcome of histologically benign conditions such as gastroesophageal reflux and esophagitis, as well as of premalignant and malignant states, ranging from the dysplasia of chronic reflux esophagitis to frank cancers. The various antireflux procedures, which are preventive of malignant transformation and are now possible videoendoscopically, do not require the use of stapling techniques. However, associated conditions such as short esophagus, fibrous stricture, or malignant transformation can be remedied by procedures in which stapling concepts are helpful.

ESOPHAGEAL PERFORATION: PRIMARY REPAIR

Esophageal perforation, which is most often the consequence of diagnostic endoluminal endoscopy and biopsy, or more rarely seen in penetrating trauma, together with usually more serious intrathoracic injuries, should be repaired primarily if it is diagnosed promptly. This repair can be temporary if the condition for which the diagnostic esophagoscopy was undertaken requires a planned major excision and reconstruction later on and if the tissues available for primary closure are healthy and free of malignancy. At times, it may be necessary to perform an emergency esophagectomy, now possible thoracoscopically, because of the presence of tumor in the site of perforation. In these patients, the esophagus is closed at the cervicothoracic inlet and above the diaphragm with transverse TA or ENDO TA staple lines. The pharynx and stomach are cleared of secretions by lateral pharyngostomy and gastrostomy aspiration drainage, and nutrition is maintained by a feeding jejunostomy (Figure IIIE-2, D to F). A planned esophageal substitute is then undertaken semielectively at a later date.

The repair is permanent if the perforation is situated in healthy tissues and if the condition for which the diagnostic procedure was undertaken or in which a penetrating trauma is responsible, does not require a second major esophageal procedure.

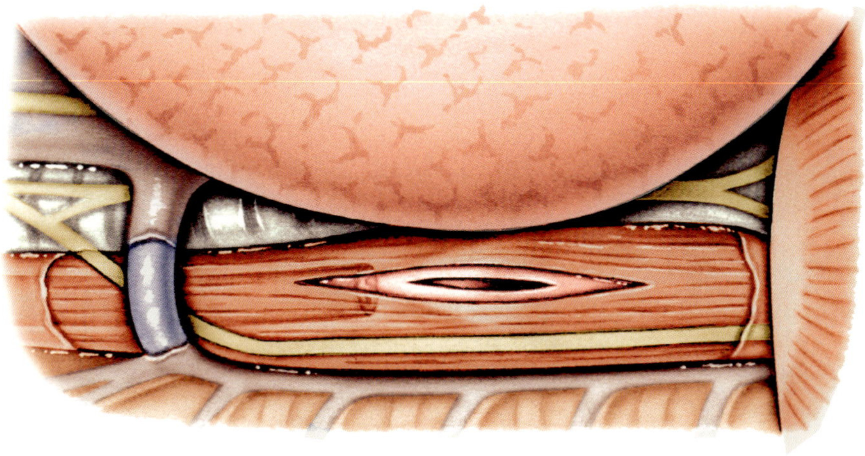

Figure III-10,A: The approach to any given perforation is decided by the hemithorax into which it occurred—in this case, it is the right side. In all repairs, opening of the mediastinal pleura from the diaphragm to the arch of the aorta and peeling of the pleura anteriorly and posteriorly, as well as debridement of infectious and necrotic material contained within the mediastinum, are mandatory. This is especially important if repair takes place after some delay, for whatever reason. A nasoesophageal tube proximal to the perforation is useful to keep the area free of nasopharyngeal secretions and to help with the diagnostic injection of methylene blue or air. After the extent of the mucosal rent has been established, the muscular wall of the esophagus is incised above and below the boundaries of the rent in order to allow the redundant mucosa to "pout" through the defect.

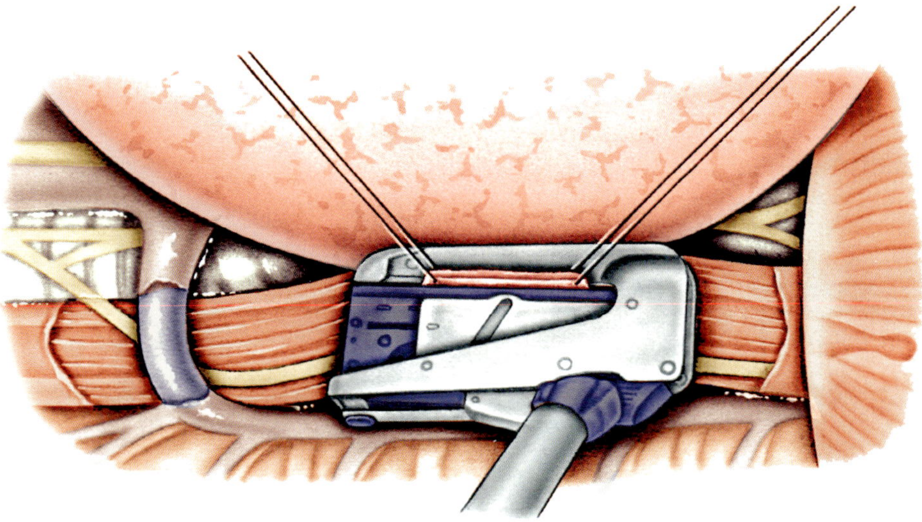

Figure III-10,B: The nasoesophageal tube is replaced with a French #48 or #52 calibrating dilator that is cautiously advanced, under direct vision, past the laceration into the stomach. Both ends and borders of the mucosal rent are elevated into and above the edges of the muscular defect with stay sutures. The inlying dilator prevents excessive narrowing of the esophageal lumen. Depending on the length of the perforation, the Roticulator 30 or 55 is placed, parallel to the axis of the esophagus, grasping between anvil and cartridge the borders of the pouting mucosa. As the instrument is closed, both borders or lips of the mucosal tear must be visible over their entire extent. The instrument is activated, achieving closure of the mucosa without the tear and wear of manual sutures on a mucosal layer only. The excess mucosa is excised along the instrument edge prior to removal of the stapler.

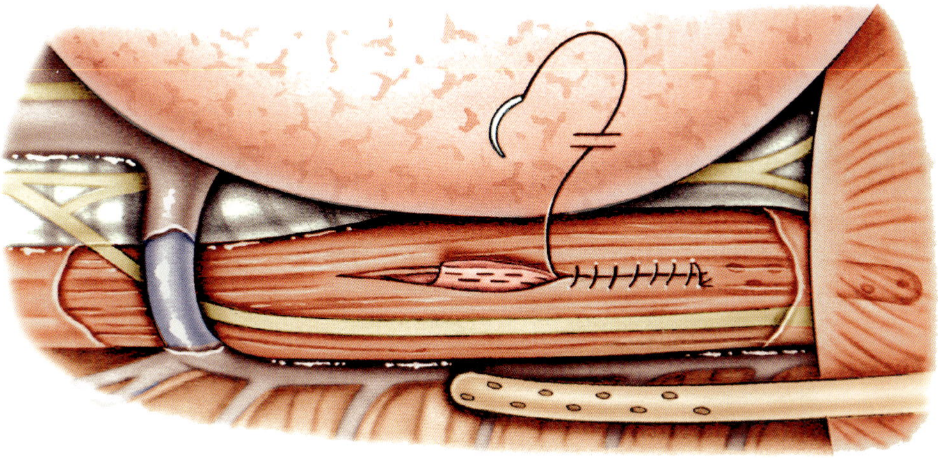

Figure III-10,C: The dilator is replaced by a nasogastric tube, and the muscular defect is closed with a running manual suture. A chest drainage tube is placed, and the incision is closed.

ESOPHAGEAL PERFORATION: T-TUBE DRAINAGE AND TEMPORARY EXCLUSION OF THE INJURED SEGMENT

In 1981, Brolin and Ravitch published results of their experimental studies on the healing of intestinal wounds sutured by manual, as well as mechanical, methods. In one of the trials, they placed linear, double staggered staple lines across the stomach, duodenum, and small bowel without transecting the respective hollow viscera distal to the closure that had totally obstructed their lumen. In all cases, they noted spontaneous restoration of transit through the stapled barriers within about 9 to 12 days, with only minimal thickening of the bowel at the staple site. Most staples were found embedded in the bowel walls, with almost complete distortion of the classical B-formation of the individual staples and straightening of their curved limbs, making the pullout from one wall of the bowel possible.

Lehur, from the Hospital Laennec and the Faculty of Medicine of the University of Nantes in France, put this finding to good use in a very original application for the treatment of complicated (e.g., Boerhaave's syndrome), at other times initially missed or neglected, esophageal perforations referred to his regional tertiary care hospital center. Having noted that the healing of esophageal wounds was impeded by both refluxing gastric acid and bacteria-carrying saliva, Lehur postulated and convincingly showed that exclusion of the injured segment would greatly bolster healing and shorten the hospital stay if the exclusion did not necessitate a second or third major operation, which, for example, a diverting pharyngostomy does require. The temporary exclusion provided by the transverse stapling of hollow viscera appeared to be an ideal solution to Lehur.

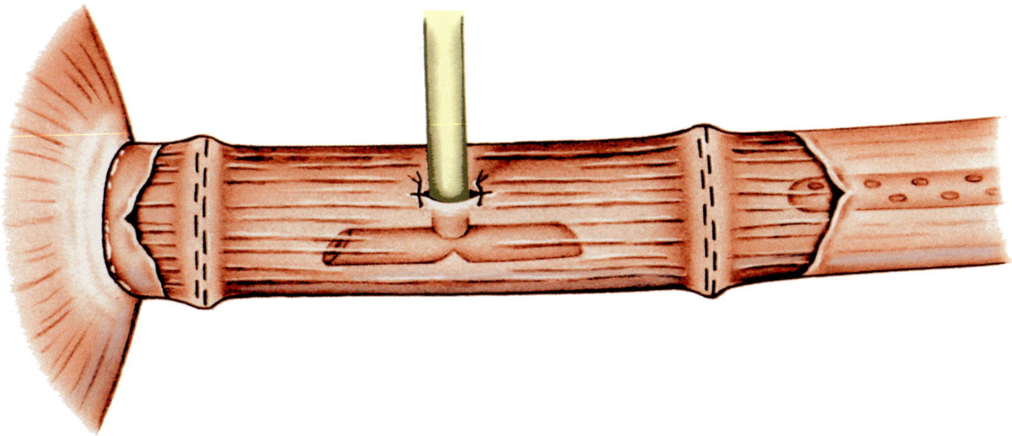

Figure III-11,A: The operation is demonstrated in the treatment of a left-sided esophageal perforation or rupture. After the requisite wide opening of the mediastinal pleura and debridement of necrosis within the mediastinum and of the esophageal wound have been accomplished, a T-tube is placed through the perforation into the esophageal lumen. The opening around the catheter is closed with full-thickness sutures. The long arm of the catheter is brought out through the lateral chest wall along a slightly dependent line to create a controlled fistula in case the traumatized esophageal tissues do not heal per primum. The esophagus is then occluded in continuity with transverse linear staple lines, above and below the perforation. A lateral pharyngostomy and a gastrostomy, both for decompression, as well as a feeding jejunostomy are then placed as shown in Figure IIIE-2, D to F. Progress in the reopening of the esophageal lumen is monitored by repeated endoluminal endoscopies, and the endoluminal drainage tube is removed after the patient has been started successfully on an oral diet and after all wounds and incisions have securely healed. In addition, pharyngostomy, gastrostomy, and jejunostomy tubes are removed in stages at that time.

ESOPHAGOGASTRECTOMY AND END-TO-SIDE ESOPHAGOGASTROSTOMY

This operation, together with adequate lymph node dissections, represents the procedure of choice for malignant lesions of the lower third of the esophagus. The dissection takes place through separate right (Ivor Lewis approach—our preference) or left thoracic and abdominal midline incisions. In the chest, the esophagus is dissected to provide a satisfactory circumferential and longitudinal tumor-free margin, proximal to the lower third lesion. Mediastinal lymph node dissection is performed "en bloc" with the specimen. The transection of the esophagus, usually in its middle third, is controlled by intraoperative histological examination to ensure a tumor-free margin. In the abdomen, lymph node dissection of the celiac axis and its branches and splenectomy are performed as indicated, together with mobilization of a generous portion of gastric fundus, "en bloc" with the thoracic specimen.

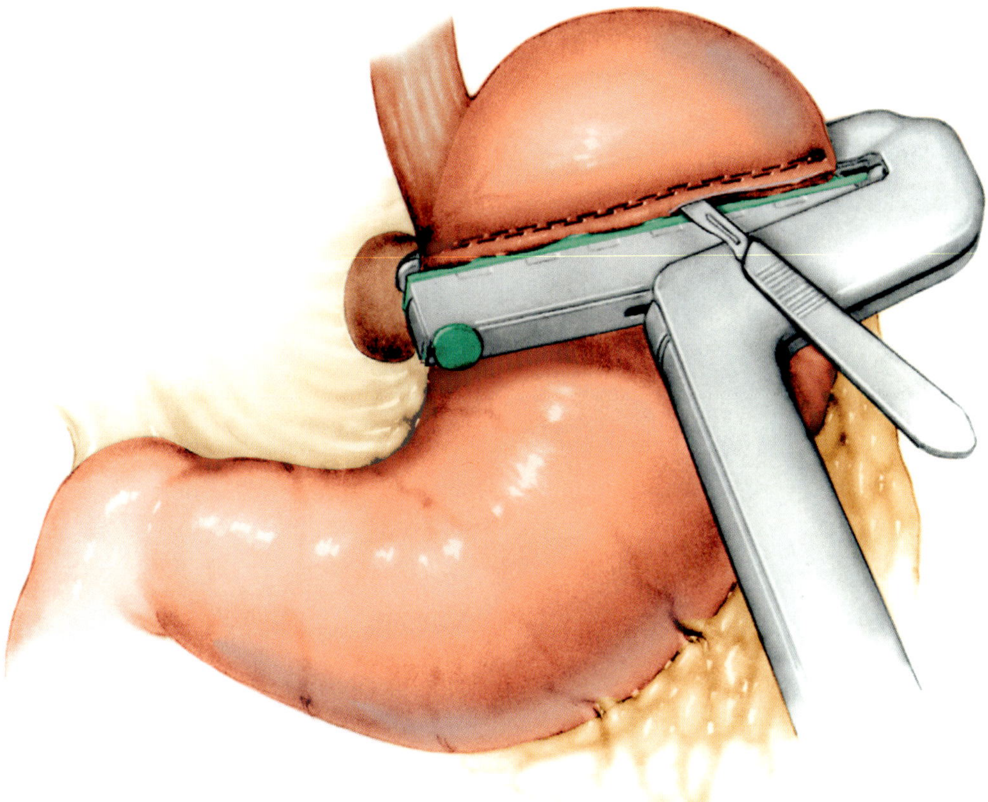

Figure III-12,A: Following mobilization of the distal esophagus and proximal stomach, the gastric fundus is stapled transversely at the level of planned resection with two applications of the TA 90 instrument. The first application is placed on the specimen side, followed by a second application distal and parallel to the previous staple line. Prior to removing the instrument used to place the second, caudad staple line, the stomach is transected along the superior edge of the TA 90 stapler.

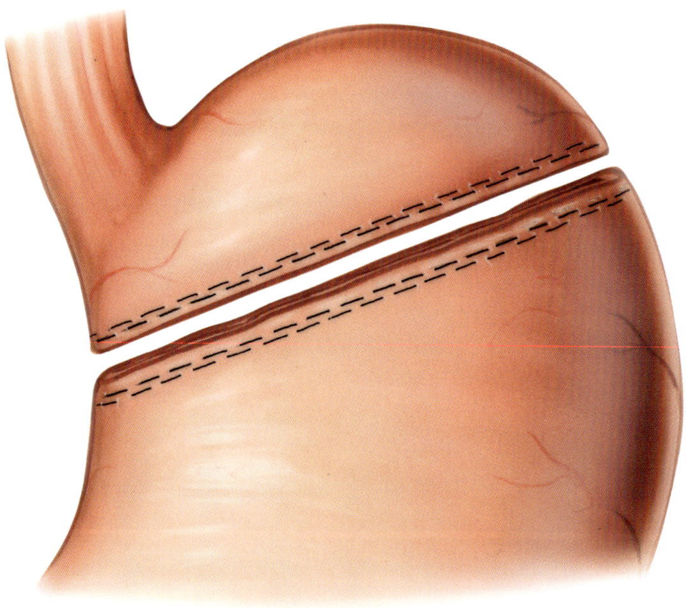

Figure III-12,B: Closure of both the remaining stomach and the specimen reduces the potential for intraperitoneal contamination.

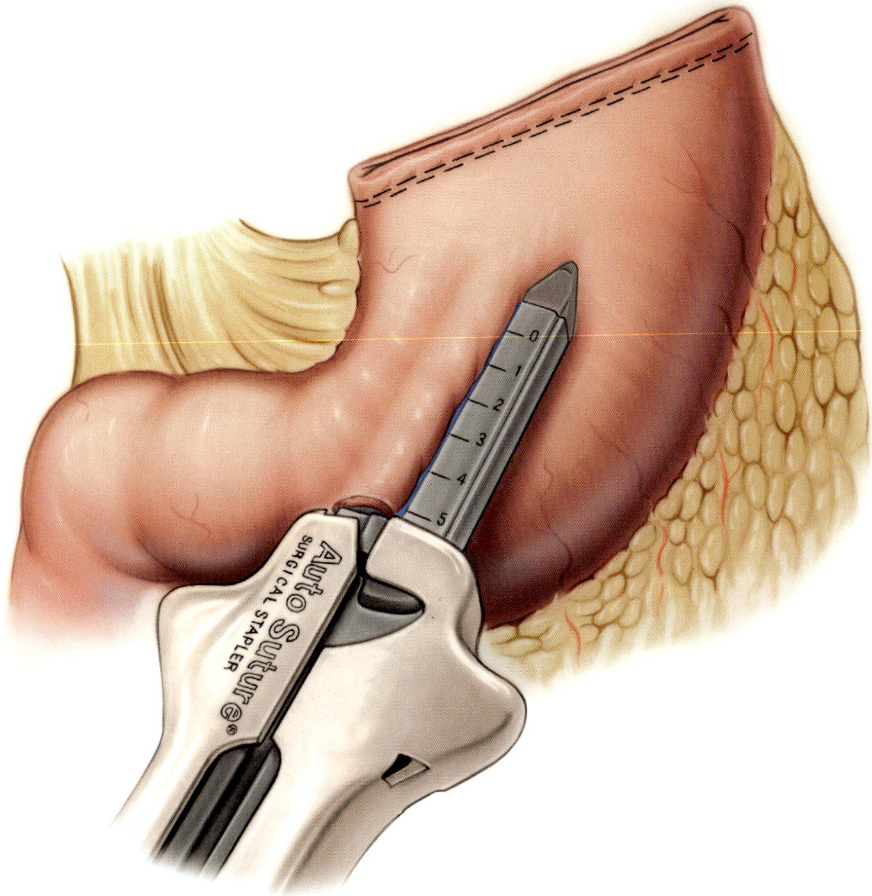

Figure III-12,C: A gastrotomy is performed with the GIA instrument. The anvil fork of the instrument is inserted into the gastric lumen through a 1 cm stab wound in the mid-to-lower third of the anterior wall of the remaining stomach at a minimum of 10 cm distal to the gastric closure. The cartridge-bearing fork is matched on the serosal surface to the intraluminal fork. The open instrument is advanced proximally over the distance that will accommodate the passage of the EEA instrument chosen for the esophagogastric anastomosis. The GIA halves are closed, the instrument is activated, and a gastrotomy with hemostatic edges is obtained.

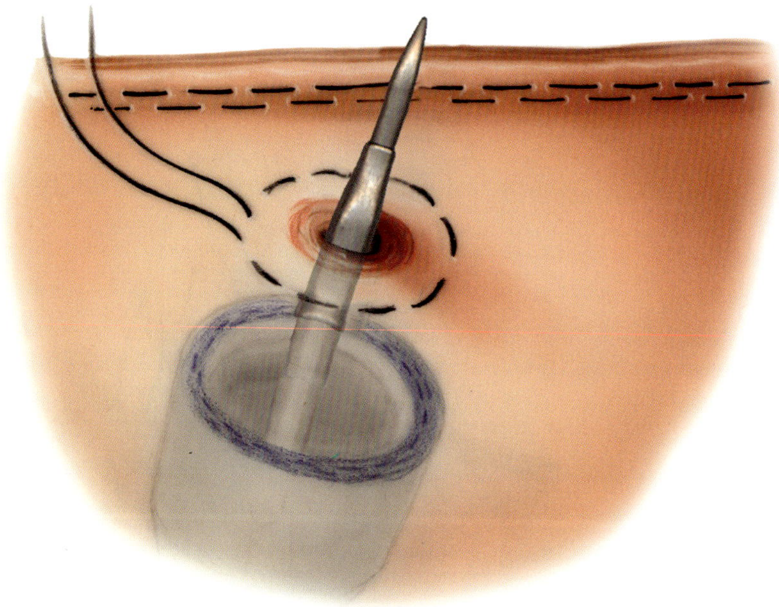

Figure III-12,D: The EEA instrument, without anvil, is inserted through the gastrotomy and positioned at the site chosen for anastomosis. The instrument is opened fully, allowing the tip of the center rod to perforate the anterior gastric wall 3 to 4 cm caudad to the stapled gastric closure. A manual purse-string suture is placed around the perforation site to prevent any serosal tearing or tissue slippage, and the suture is tied snugly, but not too tightly, around the center rod of the instrument.

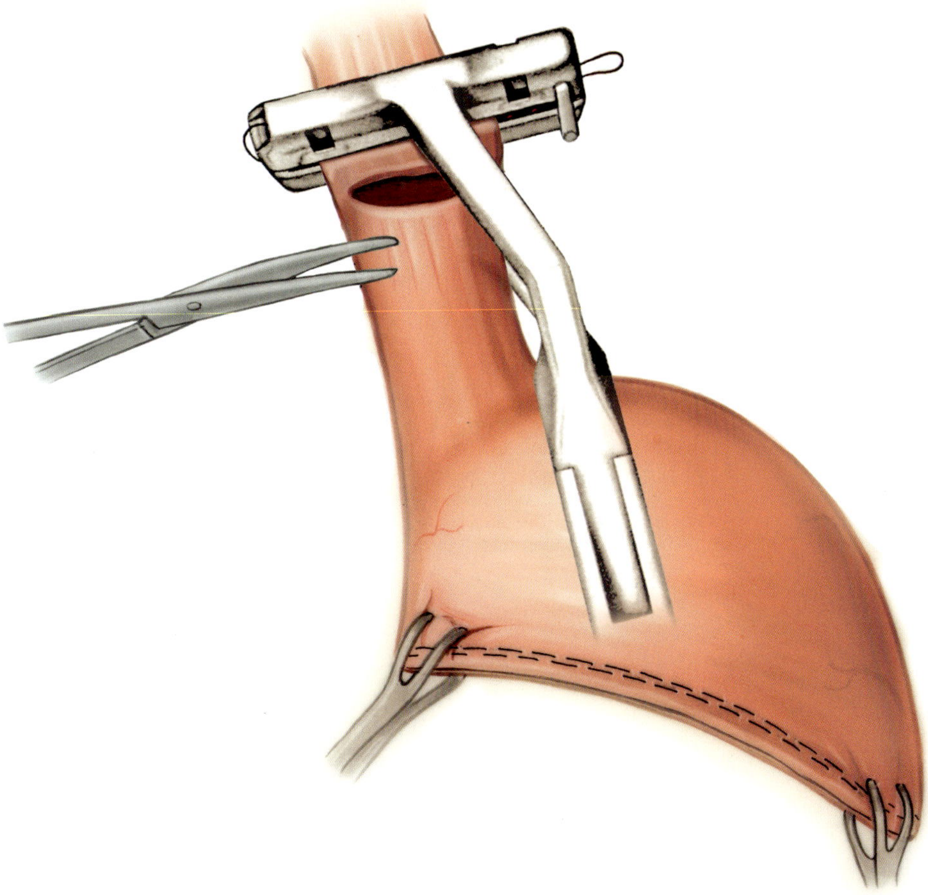

Figure III-12,E: With gentle traction on the specimen, the Purstring instrument is positioned around the esophagus just proximal to the point of resection. A purse-string suture is placed. Prior to removal of the instrument, the anterior wall of the esophagus is incised along the inferior instrument edge.

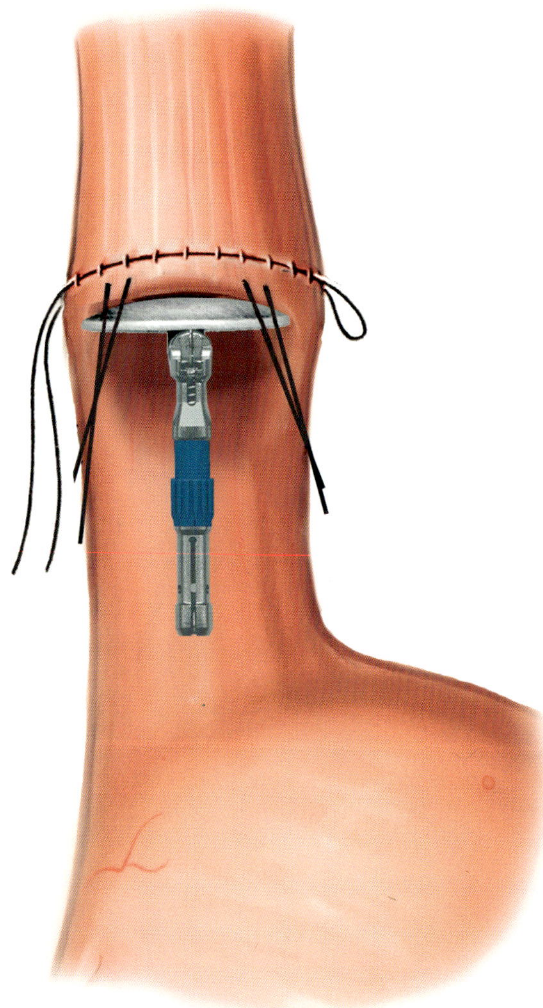

Figure III-12,F: After removing the Purstring instrument, stay sutures are placed at both ends of the transverse incision. While holding up the stay sutures of the anterior wall of the esophagus, to open its lumen, and exerting gentle downward traction on the specimen, the anvil of the EEA instrument is inserted into the esophagus.

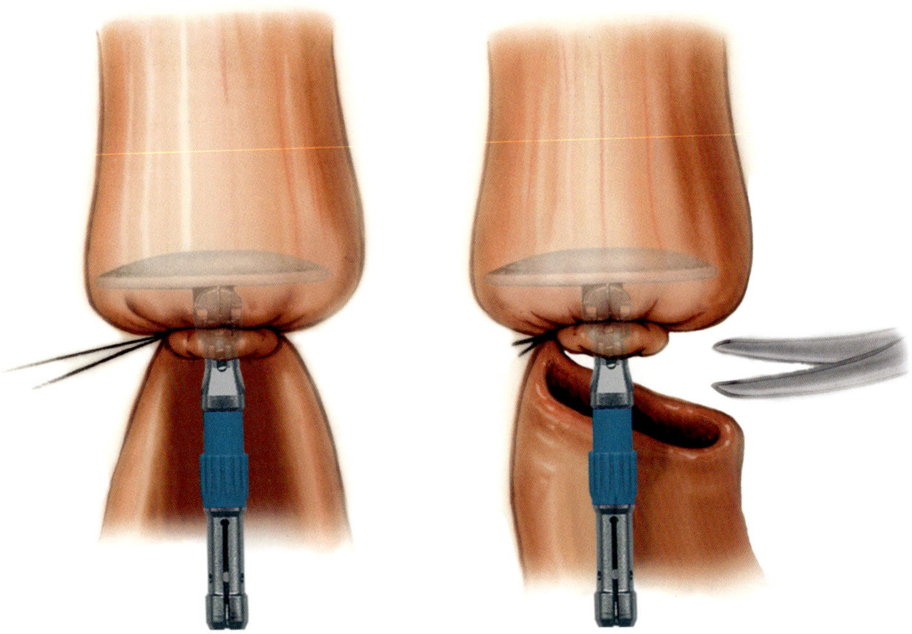

Figure III-12,G,H: The purse-string suture is tied firmly around the anvil shaft, and the posterior wall of the esophagus is transected, taking care not to compromise the integrity of the circular closure. The resection of the esophagogastric specimen is now complete.

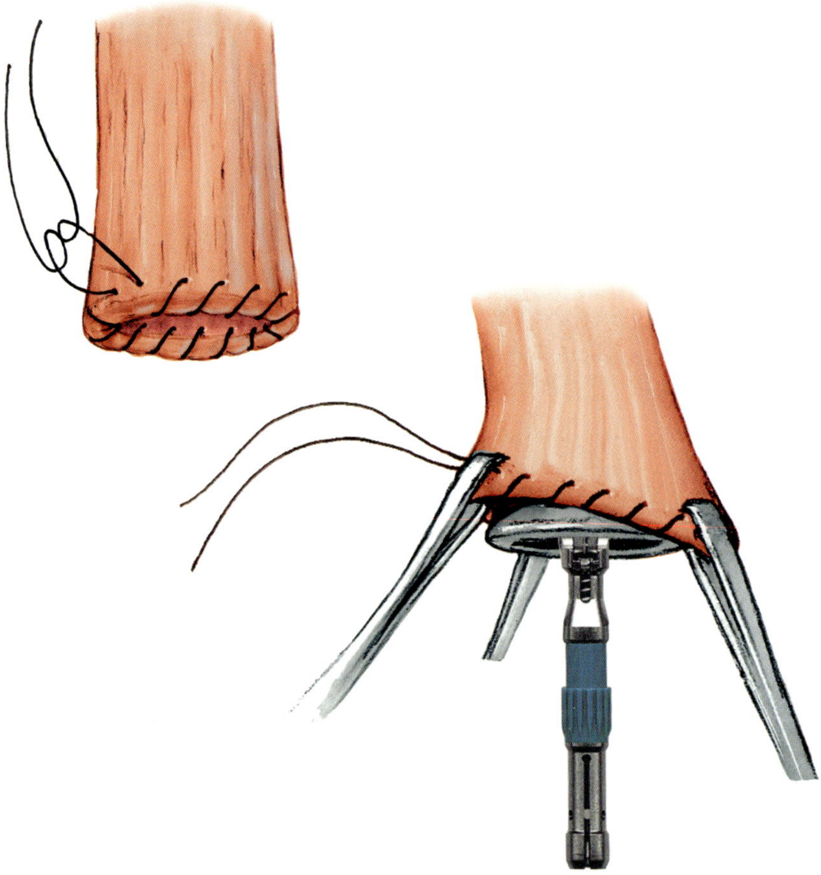

Figure III-12,I,J: If placement of the Purstring instrument is onerous because of limited exposure, the esophagus may be transected completely in a first step. The specimen is removed to free up space. The purse-string suture is then placed with a manual 2-0, monofilament, over-and-over full-thickness whipstitch, rounding the entire circumference of the esophageal stump, starting and ending at close points on the serosa. With the aid of three Allis clamps or stay sutures, placed equidistantly and holding open the rim of the esophagus, the anvil is advanced into the esophageal lumen and the purse-string suture is tied firmly around the anvil shaft.

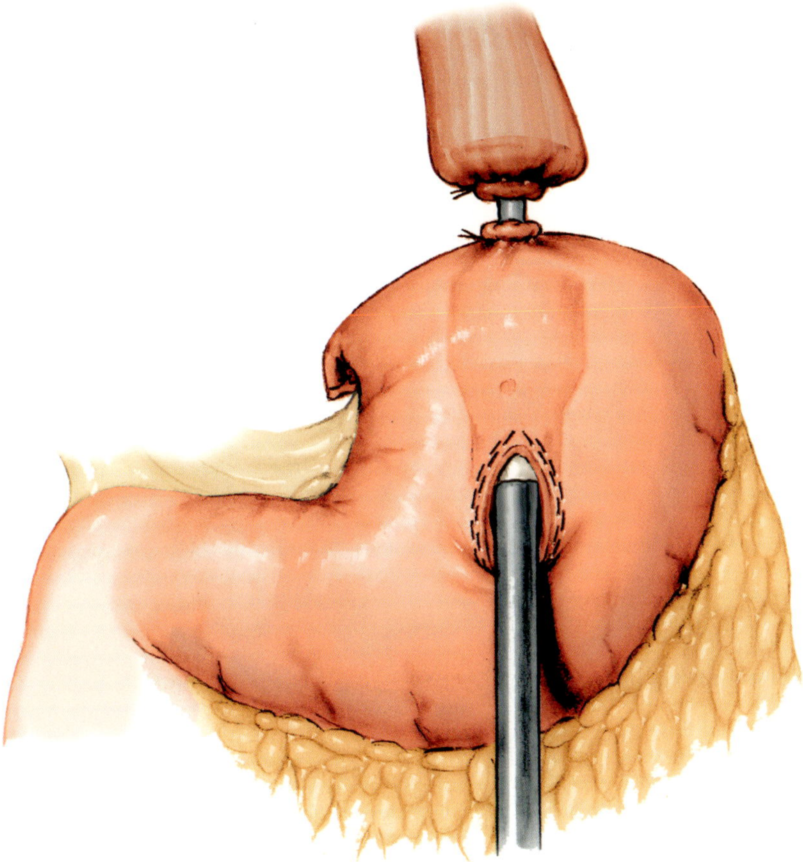

Figure III-12,K: The anvil shaft and center rod of the EEA instrument are mated, and the instrument is closed, taking care that the tissue is snug against the cartridge and anvil and that no extraneous tissue is incarcerated between the stomach and esophagus.

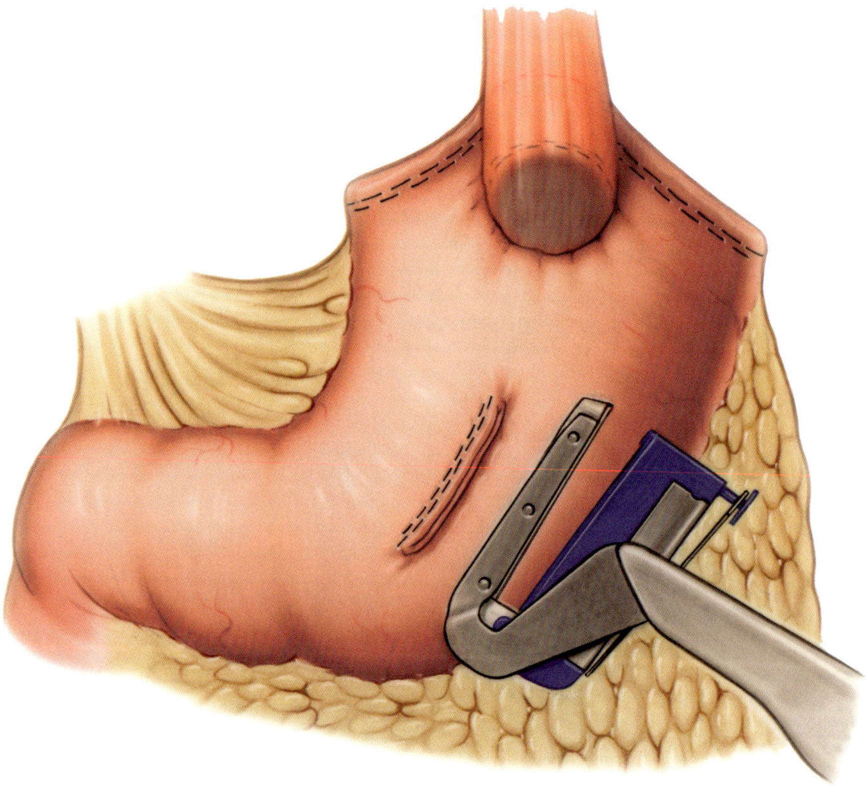

Figure III-12,L: Following completion of the end-to-side esophagogastrostomy, the circular stapling instrument is removed, the completeness of excised tissue "donuts" and the integrity of the anastomosis are verified, and the anterior gastrotomy is closed with a linear stapler.

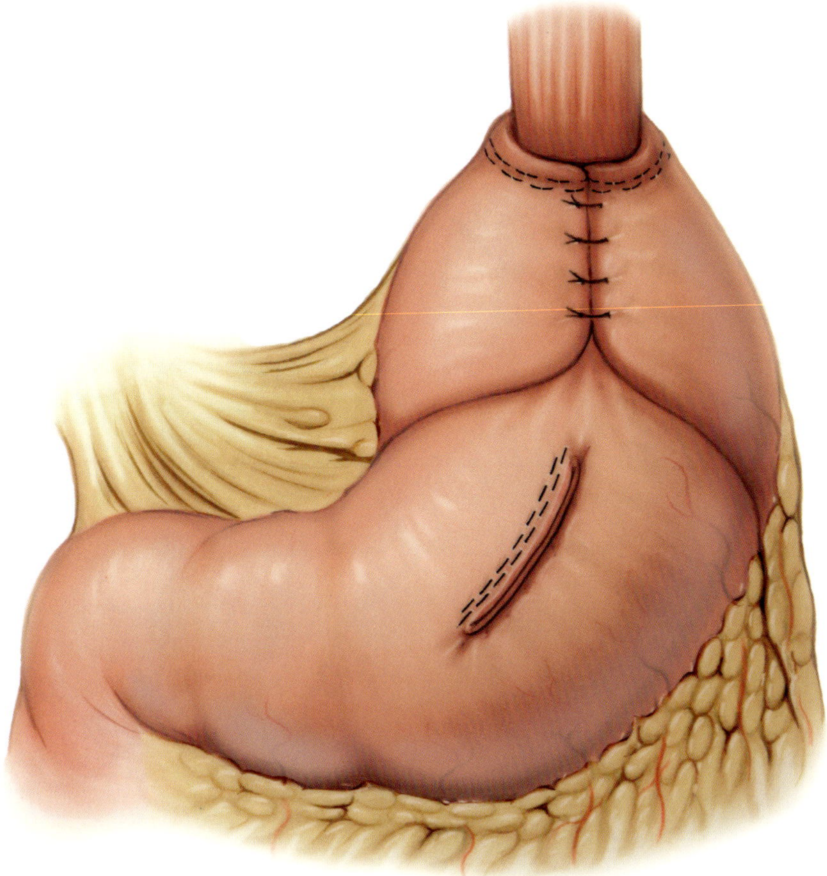

Figure III-12,M: If the remaining stomach is wide and reaches the anastomosis with some redundancy in width and length, it is wrapped and sutured around the anastomosis in a modified Nissen mode to provide an antireflux mechanism to what is essentially a wide open conduit for acid or alkaline gastric juices to inundate and irritate the esophagus. An additional advantage of this gastric plication is the protection offered the anastomosis by coverage of the thick plicated gastric wall.

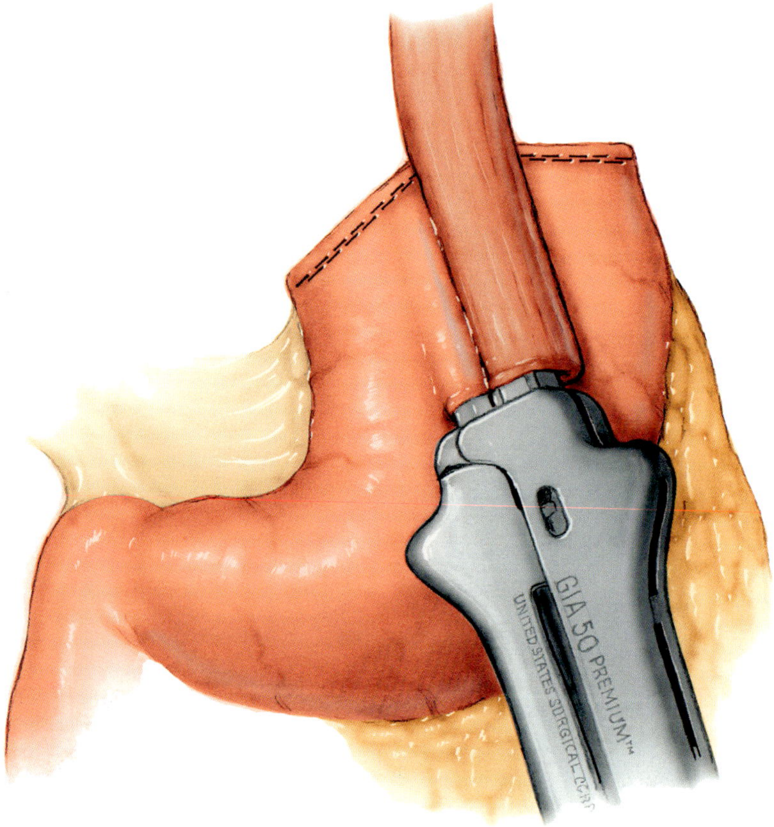

Figure III-12,N: Radical esophagogastrectomy should never be hostage to a single reconstructive technique of digestive tract continuity since the circumstances and difficulties encountered in each patient may require excisional strategies that would create a vacuum if only a single pattern of anatomical restoration was available. One alternative, of several proposed in this text, is esophagogastrostomy performed using the GIA instrument. For this anastomosis, the esophagus must be elevated from its bed over the length of the GIA instrument and placed on the anterior surface of the stomach. A 1 cm stab wound is made in the midanterior wall of the gastric remnant approximately 6 to 8 cm distal to the stapled gastric closure. The anvil fork of the GIA instrument is placed into the lumen of the stomach and the cartridge fork into the open-ended lumen of the esophagus. The tissue is evenly aligned on the forks of the instrument, which is then closed and activated.

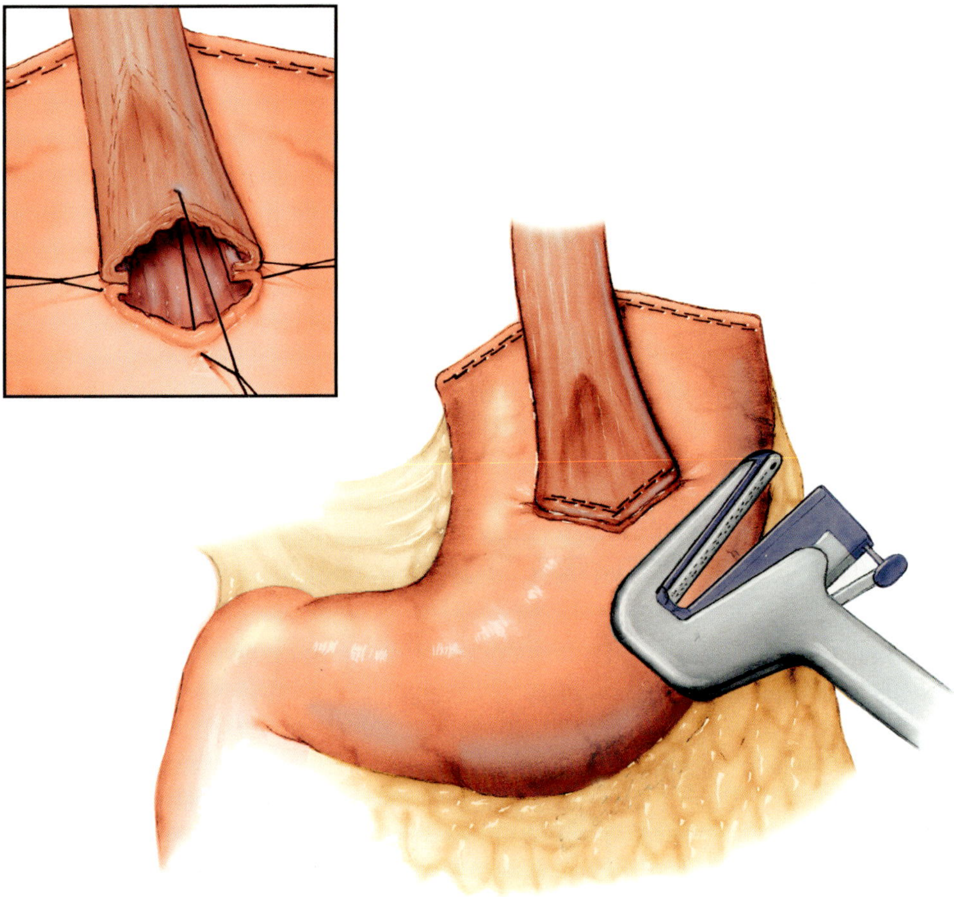

Figure III-12,O: After removal of the instrument, the anastomosis is inspected for hemostasis. The linear staple lines joining the esophagus and stomach are held at the 3 o'clock and 9 o'clock positions of the now common GIA placement site by two everting stay sutures. A third suture is placed through the midpoints of the common opening, triangulating the circular rim of this opening as the midpoint suture is pulled tight.

Figure III-12,P: As traction is placed on two consecutive stay sutures (e.g., 3 o'clock and 6 o'clock positions, 6 o'clock and 9 o'clock positions), the convex esophageal rim is placed against the concave gastric rim, forming semicircular pouting (everting) lips. These lips of esophageal wall above and gastric wall below are sutured in a cuneiform fashion with two applications of the TA 30 instrument, ensuring that all tissue layers and the ends of the previous placed staple lines are incorporated within these linear closures. The excess tissue is excised along the free edge of the linear stapler after each application, while preserving the midpoint stay suture between the first and the second application. This ensures complete closure of the entire semicircular pouting (everted) esophagogastric rims.

ESOPHAGOGASTRECTOMY WITH COMBINED ESOPHAGOGASTROSTOMY AND PYLOROPLASTY

A drainage procedure of a large gastric remnant may appear desirable, especially after truncal vagotomy usually associated with radical esophagogastrectomy. Early in our experience, we performed a pyloromyotomy as a matter of routine. However, we learned with experience that emptying of the residual stomach does resume a normal rhythm about 2 to 3 months after operation and that the routine use of an additional operative step is not indicated. If, however, a pyloroplasty is desirable according to the surgeon's judgment, it can be integrated into the esophagogastrostomy if stapling techniques are used for both operative steps.

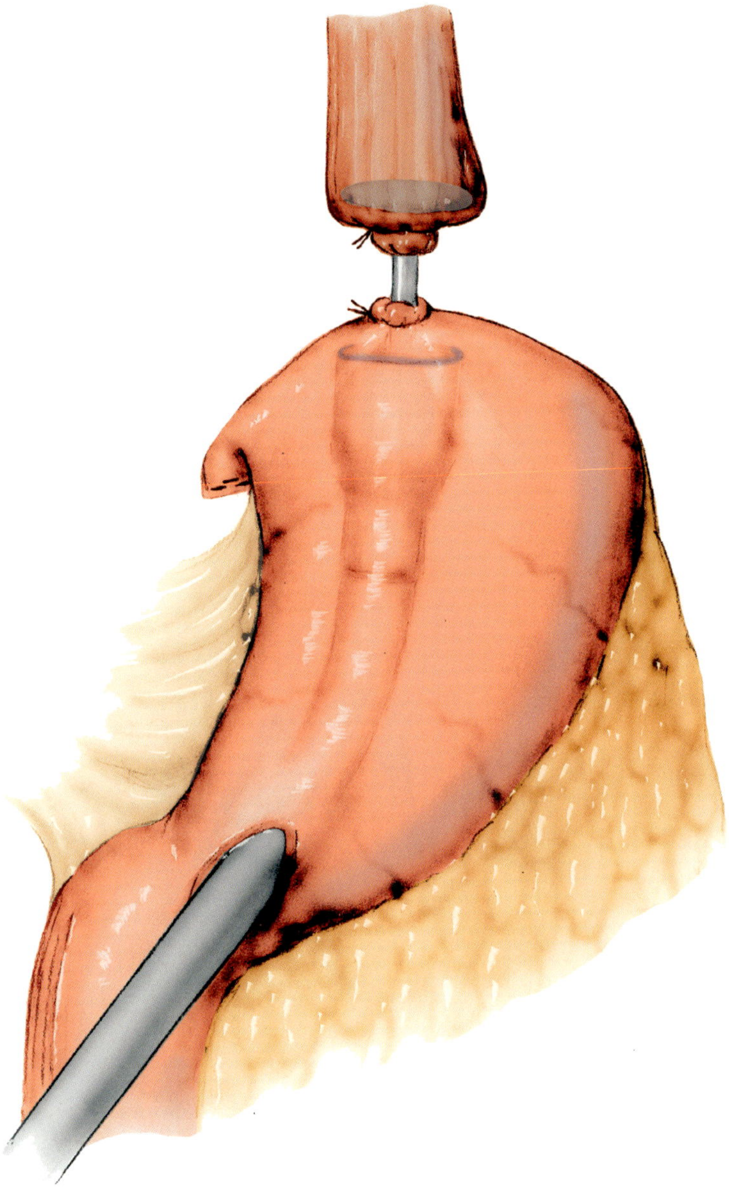

Figure III-13,A: The esophagogastrectomy is begun as described in Figure III-12,A,B. A longitudinal incision of 4 cm in the long axis of the stomach and duodenum is made across the pylorus. The EEA instrument, without anvil, is inserted through this incision and advanced to the site for the esophagogastrostomy. The procedure is then continued and accomplished as described in Figure III-12, D to K.

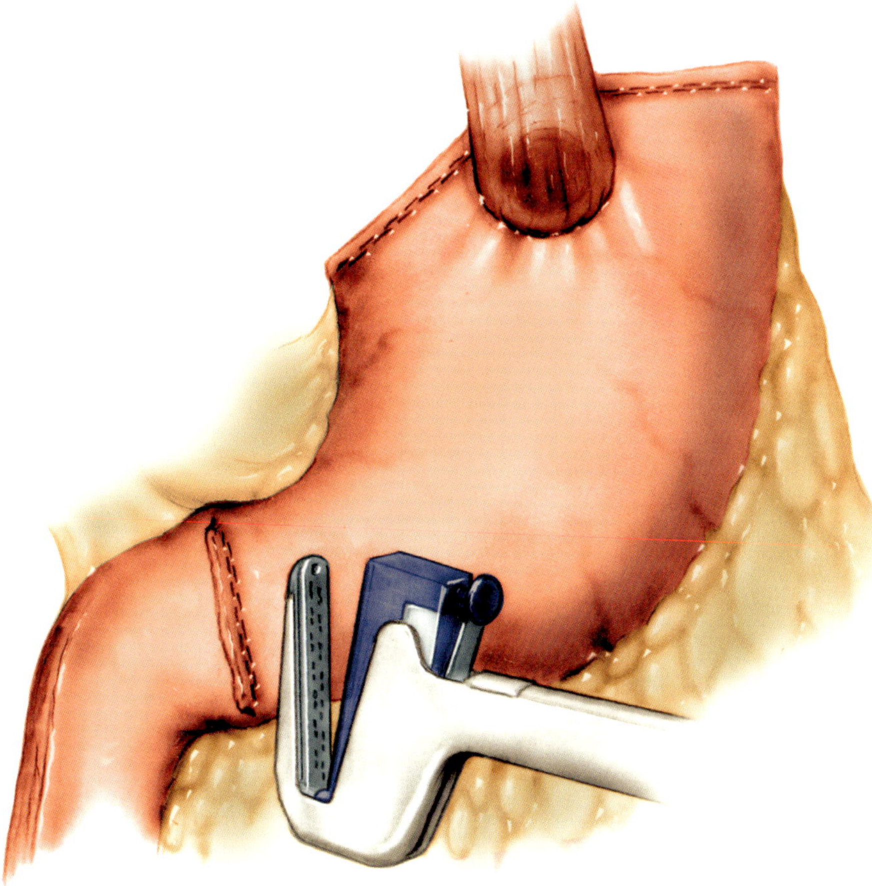

Figure III-13,B: Following completion of the end-to-side anastomosis, the circular stapling instrument is removed, and the completeness of the tissue "donuts" and purse-string sutures and the integrity of the anastomosis are examined. The pyloric incision is closed transversely with the linear stapler in the classical Heineke-Mikulicz mode.

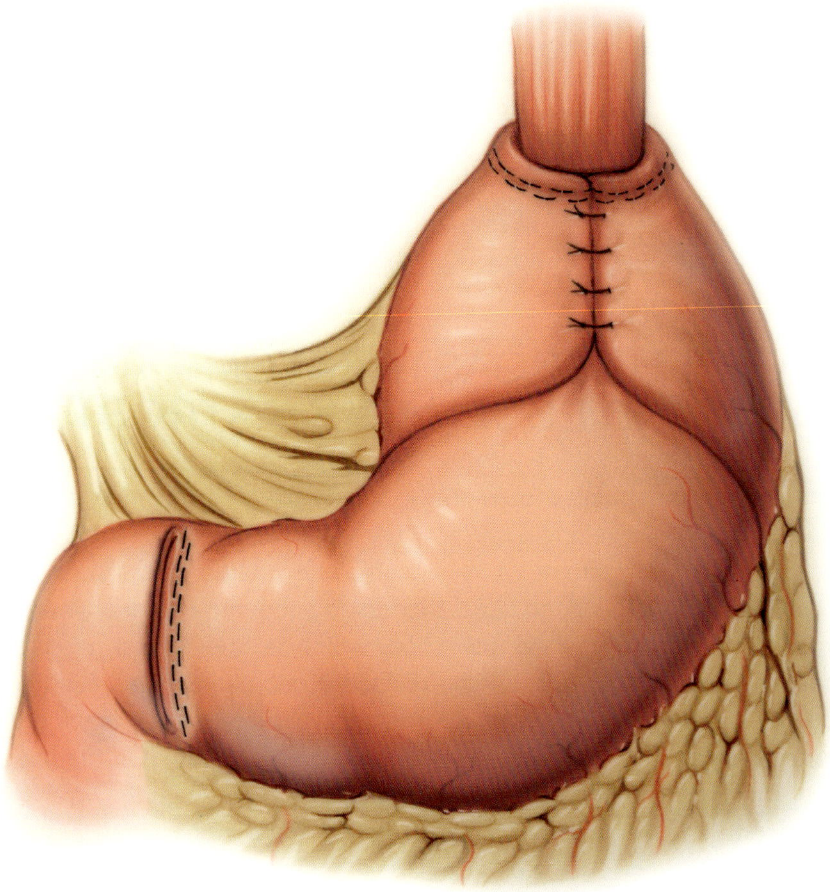

Figure III-13,C: Once again, plication of the proximal stomach can be performed for security and to provide an antireflux mechanism.

ESOPHAGOGASTRECTOMY AND END-TO-END ESOPHAGOGASTROSTOMY

For patients with chronic obstructive pulmonary disease (COPD) who require postoperative mechanical ventilation and positive end-expiratory pressure (PEEP), the space behind and above the end-to-side esophagogastrostomy may accumulate gastric secretions, especially if a circumferential gastric plication has been used. Increased pulmonary parenchymal pressures may cause the progressively increasing fluid collection, which is due to lack of drainage into the stomach, to rise to levels that can rupture the distended stomach in this blind space between anastomosis and transverse gastric closure. In order to avoid this mishap in patients with COPD, an end-to-end anastomosis that eliminates altogether any blind nooks and crannies is preferred. In addition, by placing the anastomosis through the greater curvature corner, the remaining stomach can be elongated diagonally without risk and therefore can reach higher levels in the hemithorax.

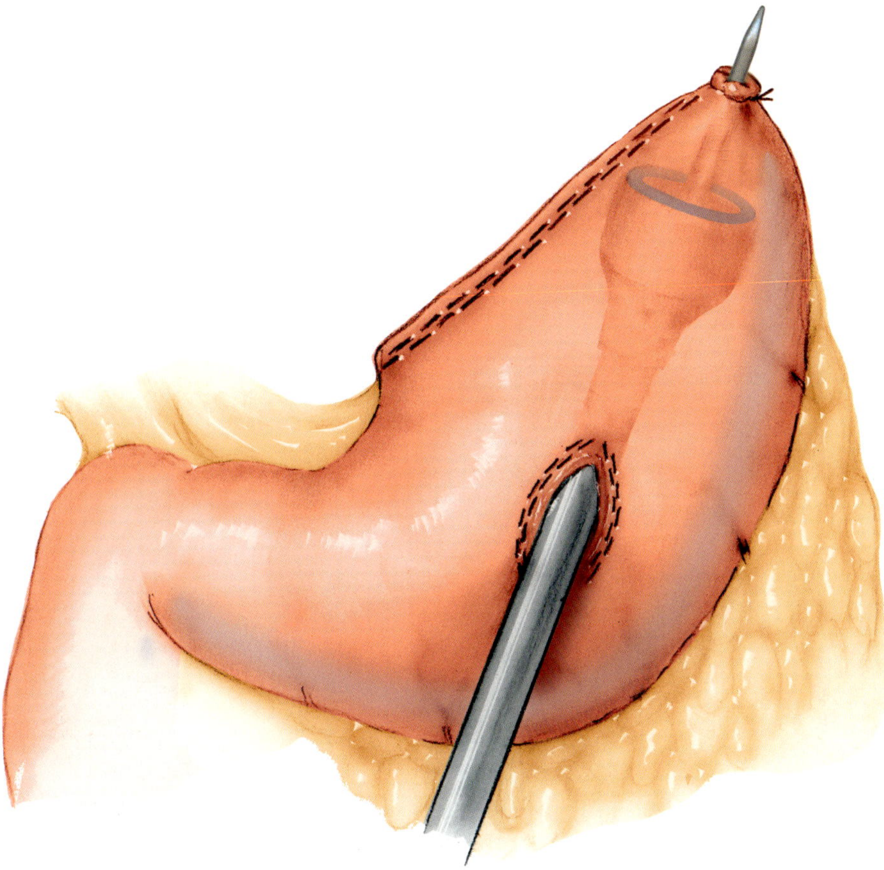

Figure III-14,A: The esophagogastrectomy and gastrotomy are performed as described in Figure III-12, A to C. The EEA instrument, without anvil, is inserted through the gastrotomy and positioned at the greater curvature corner of the gastric closure for anastomosis. The instrument is opened fully, allowing the tip to perforate the gastric wall, and a manual purse-string suture is placed and secured around the center rod of the instrument.

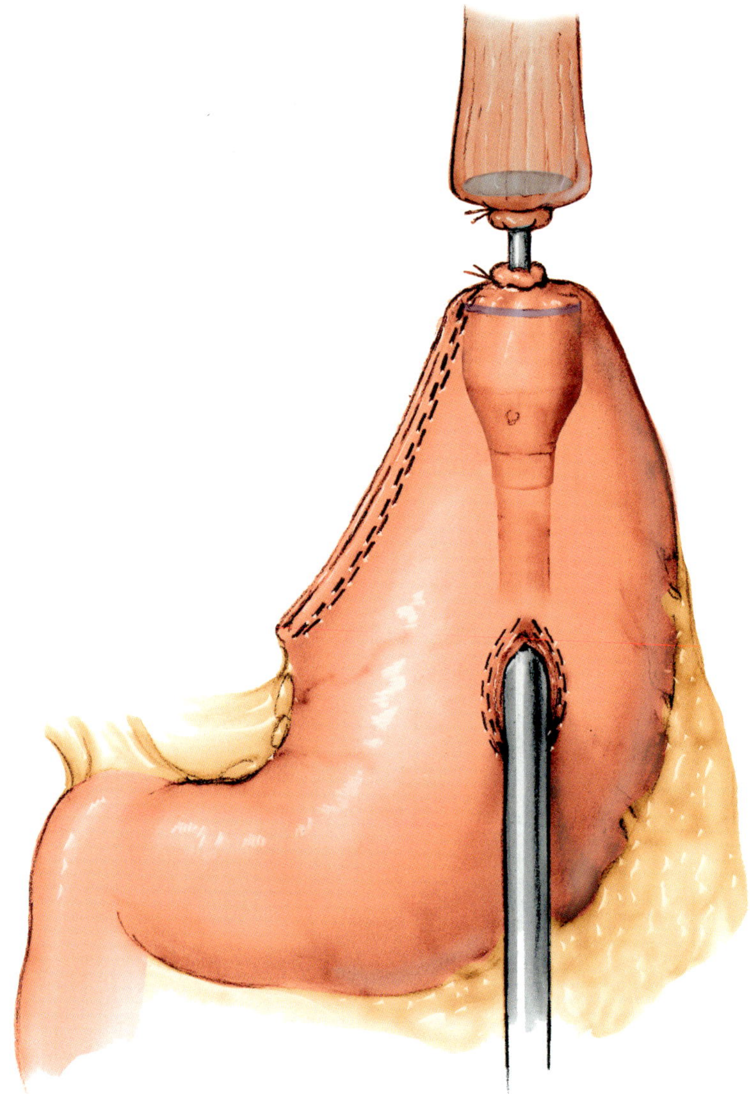

Figure III-14,B: The esophagus is fitted with a purse-string suture, the anvil is placed inside the esophageal lumen, and the purse-string suture is tied, as shown in Figure III-12, E to K.

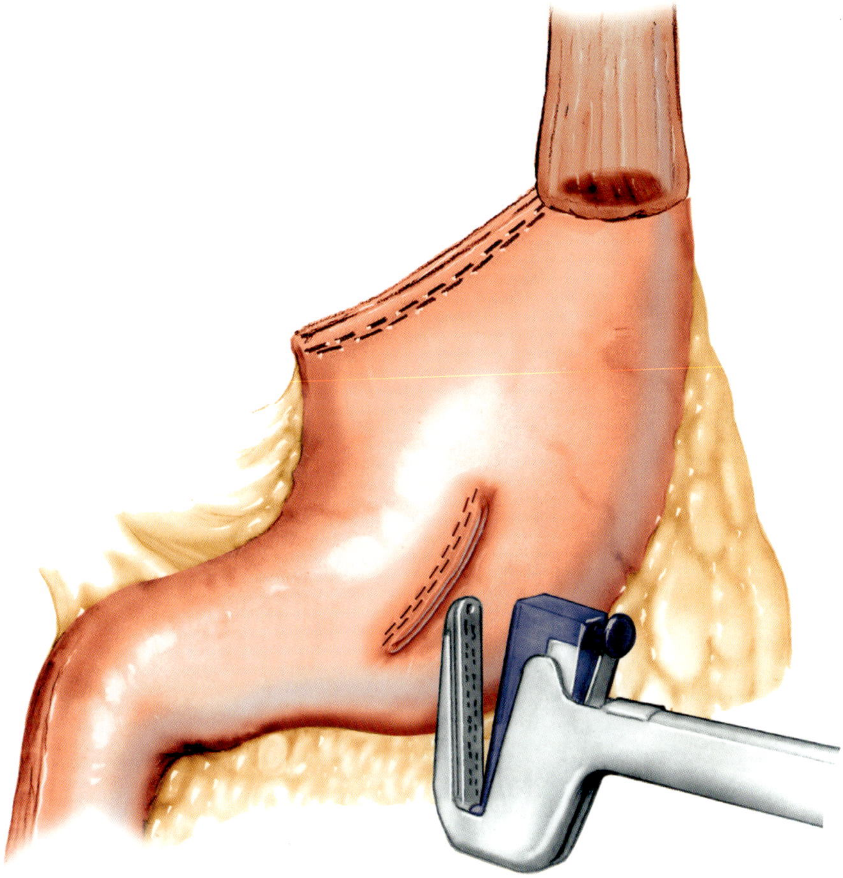

Figure III-14,C: Following completion of the end-to-end esophagogastrostomy, the circular stapling instrument is removed, the completeness of the tissue "donuts" and integrity of the anastomosis are checked, and the anterior gastrotomy is closed with a linear stapler.

TRANSDIAPHRAGMATIC ESOPHAGOGASTRECTOMY, CREATION OF A WIDE ISOPERISTALTIC GASTRIC TUBE, AND END-TO-END OR END-TO-SIDE ESOPHAGOGASTROSTOMY

For this distal esophagectomy and extended proximal gastrectomy that was initially undertaken through a left thoracotomy, the dissection takes place first in the mediastinum, then through the diaphragm into the upper abdomen. A collar of diaphragm is removed at the hiatus, together with the specimen. Since the tumor straddles both mediastinum and abdomen, the dissection is completed below the diaphragm through a separate midline incision. It includes safe margins above and below the tumor of the GE junction, appropriate lymph node dissections, and splenectomy, if indicated. The laparotomy also facilitates the placement of the EEA anastomotic instrument into the gastric tube and helps in carrying it across the hiatus into the left chest.

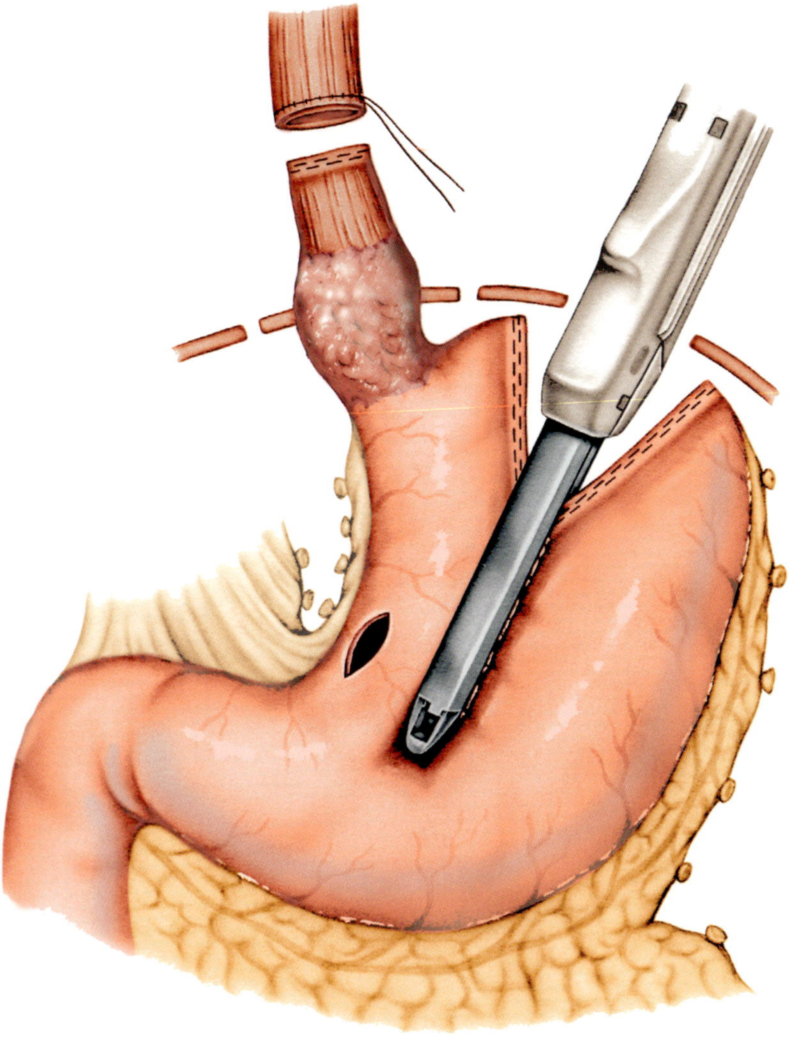

Figure III-15,A: The distal esophageal part of the specimen is closed with the TA instrument to reduce the risk of contamination and spread of intraluminal tumor cells. The proximal esophagus is fitted with a purse-string suture. A wide gastric tube is created from above, downward with serial applications of the GIA instrument. The gastrotomy for the introduction of the EEA instrument is established caudally into the future specimen.

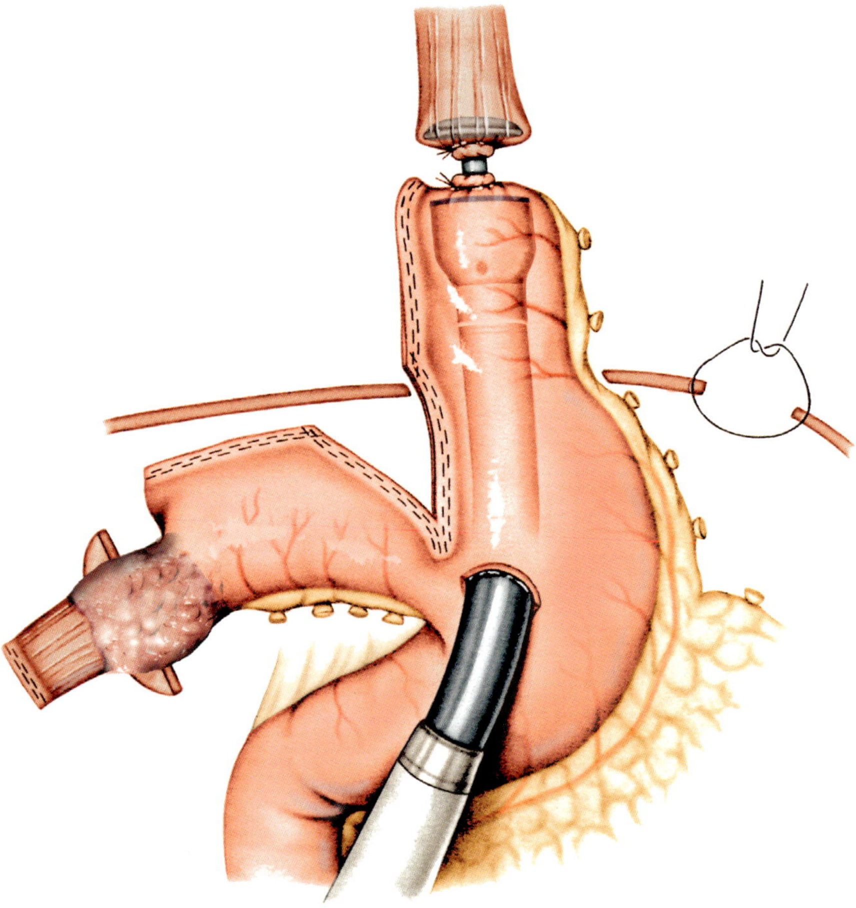

Figure III-15,B: The anvil of the EEA instrument is placed into the esophagus and the purse-string suture is tied securely around its shaft. The temporary remaining junction between specimen and stomach is closed with a tape to prevent tumor spillage (not shown in the illustration). The EEA instrument, without anvil, is introduced through the previously established gastrotomy at the remaining attachment of the specimen to the middle-lower third of the gastric body and is advanced to the site for anastomosis. With the leverage provided by the instrument, the gastric tube is carried and elevated through the hiatus into the left chest. The tip, spearheading the center rod, is advanced through the gastric wall at the planned anastomotic site, and a manual purse-string suture is placed and tied around the center rod. The anvil shaft and center rod are joined, and the instrument is closed and activated, performing the end-to-end esophagogastrostomy.

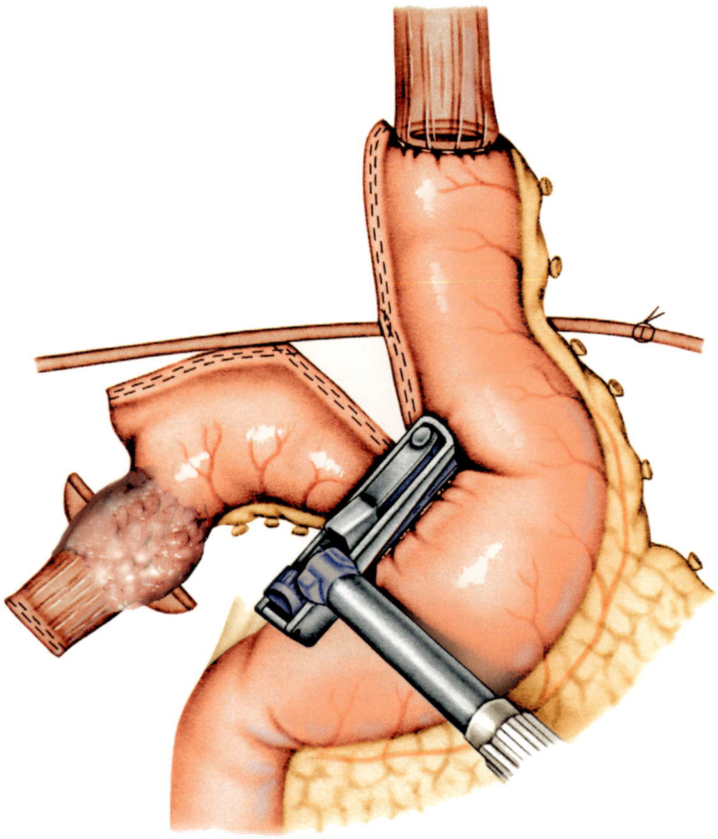

Figure III-15,C: Following completion of the anastomosis, removal of the EEA instrument, and inspection of the stoma, the specimen, including the gastrotomy, is excised peripheral to a linear staple closure. The incision in the tendinous portion of the diaphragm is repaired.

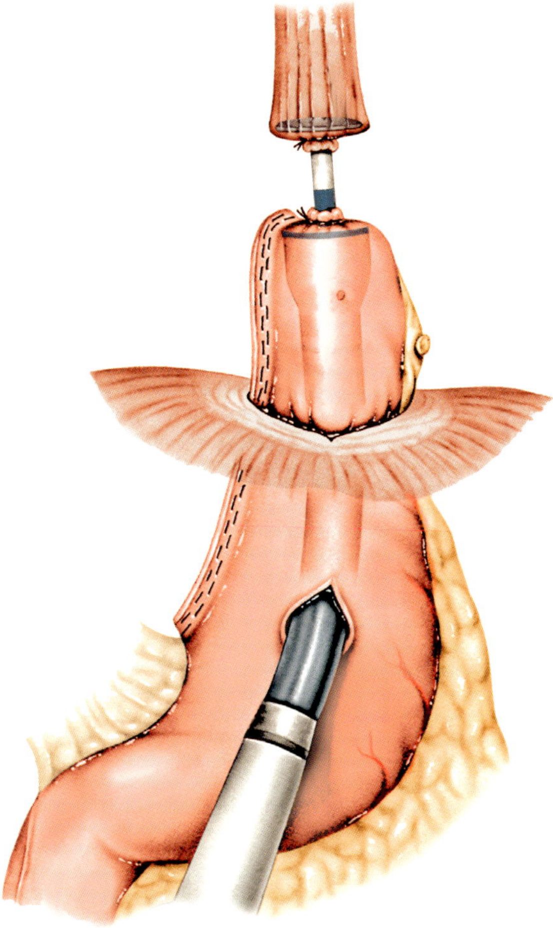

Figure III-15,D: Alternatively, the specimen may be removed first and the anastomosis performed with the EEA instrument advanced through a separate gastrotomy in the anterior wall of the wide lower body of the stomach. This gastrotomy will be closed with a linear stapler as in Figure III-12,L. In all cases where the gastric resection is performed with the GIA instrument, a running suture is used to reinforce the staple closure on the patient side (Figure III-16,C).

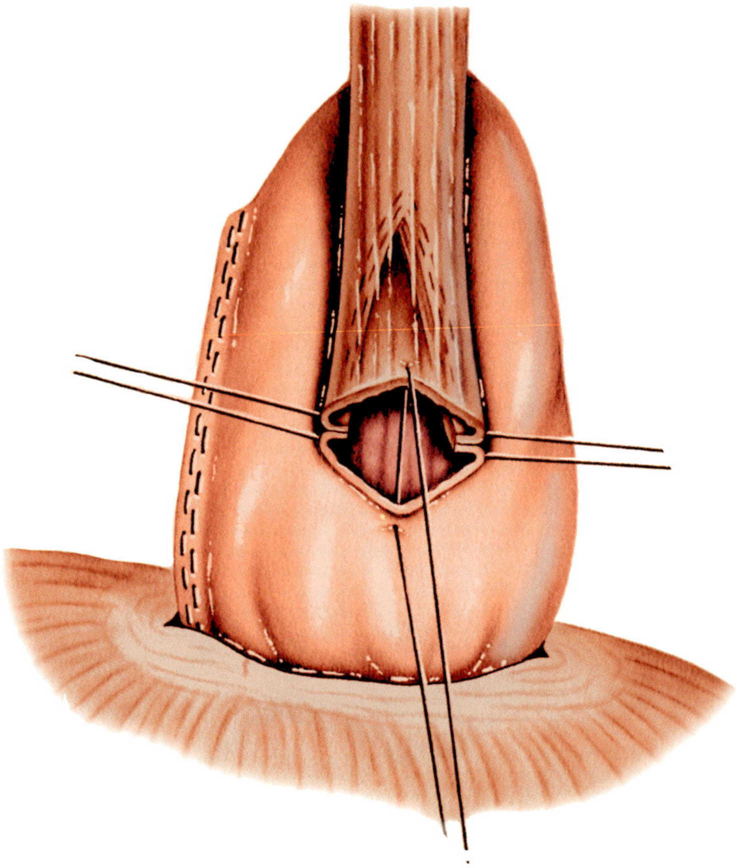

Figure III-15,E: If the proximal gastrectomy includes a safe, tumor-free portion of fundus, as well as a moderate strip of lesser curvature to elongate the resulting wider gastric tube, an end-to-side esophagogastrostomy can be constructed with the GIA and TA instruments, as in Figure III-12,N. The common GIA introduction site is prepared for closure as in Figure III-12,O, by placing three equidistant stay sutures from the esophageal rim to the gastric rim.

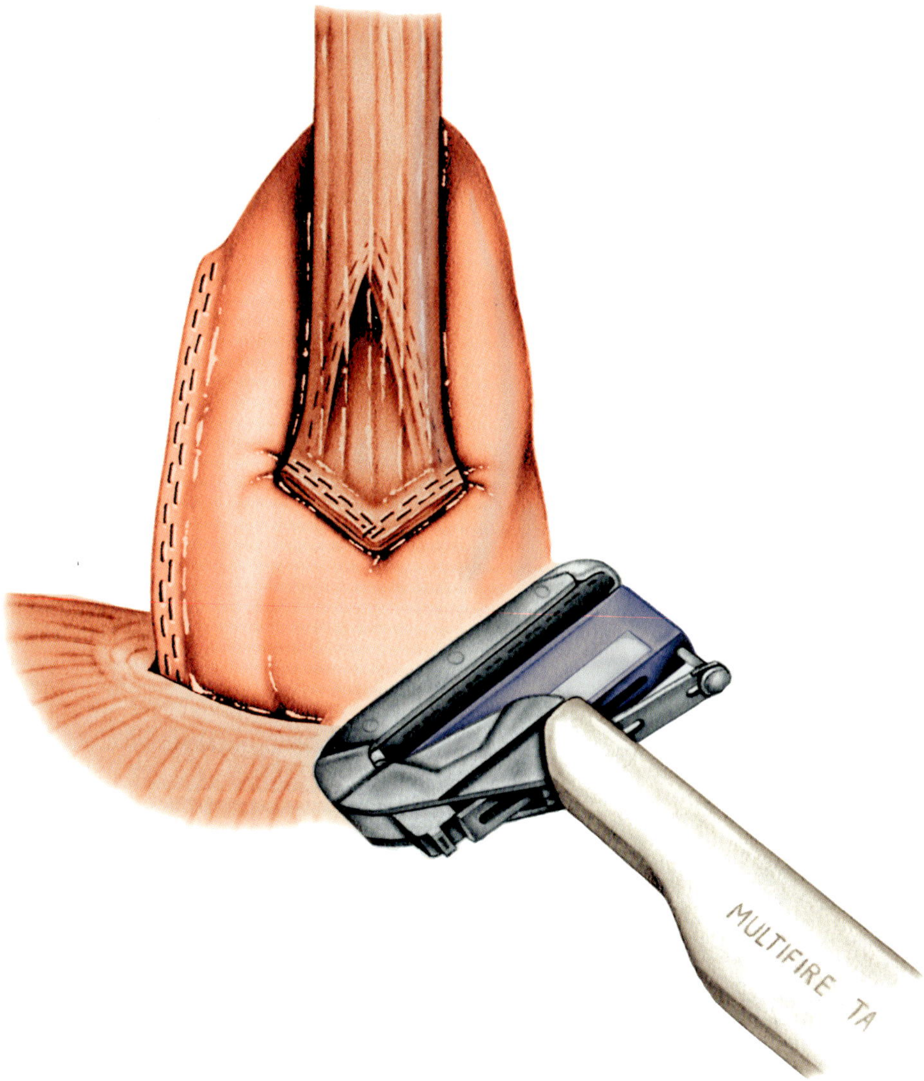

Figure III-15,F: By holding up two consecutive sutures at a time, the open circumference is transformed into two linear triangulating halves. Each half esophagogastric double rim is closed with a linear stapling instrument, mucosa-to-mucosa, taking care to incorporate all tissue layers. The staple lines overlap anteriorly in a triangular fashion and at both lateral angles with the anastomotic GIA lines.

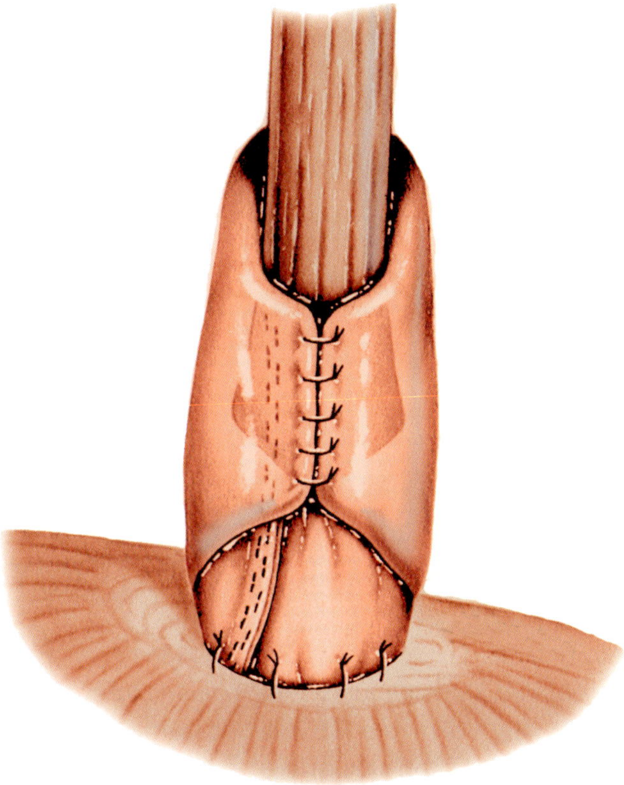

Figure III-15,G: A gastric wrap, if possible, is manually sutured around the anastomosis for security and to provide an antireflux mechanism.

EXTENDED ESOPHAGOGASTRECTOMY, CREATION OF A NARROW ISOPERISTALTIC GASTRIC TUBE, AND END-TO-END ESOPHAGOGASTROSTOMY

Distal esophagectomy and extended proximal gastrectomy with lymphadenectomy as indicated by staging, followed by intrathoracic, transhiatal esophagogastric tube anastomosis, are performed in patients with tumors extending below the GE junction, where a more radical excision of the proximal cardia, fundus, and body of the stomach is required. This technique can be employed through either right or left thoracotomy and a separate laparotomy.

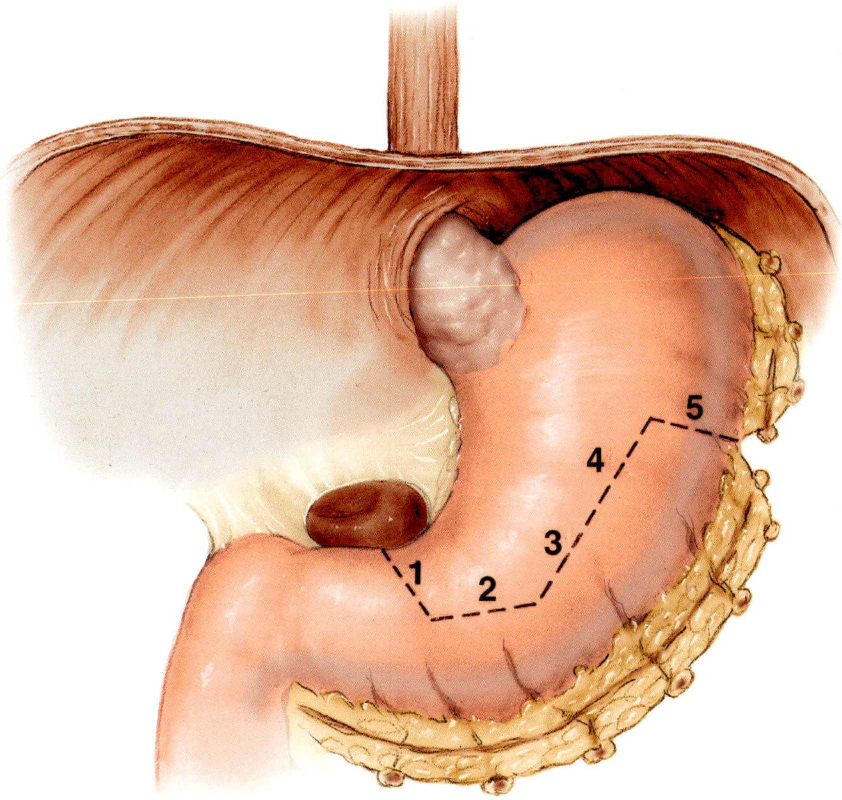

Figure III-16,A: The lower esophagus and the stomach are mobilized, leaving the gastroepiploic arcade intact for vascularization of the gastric tube. The upper half of the stomach is removed together with a wide excision of the lower, lesser curvature, resulting in a narrow isoperistaltic gastric tube.

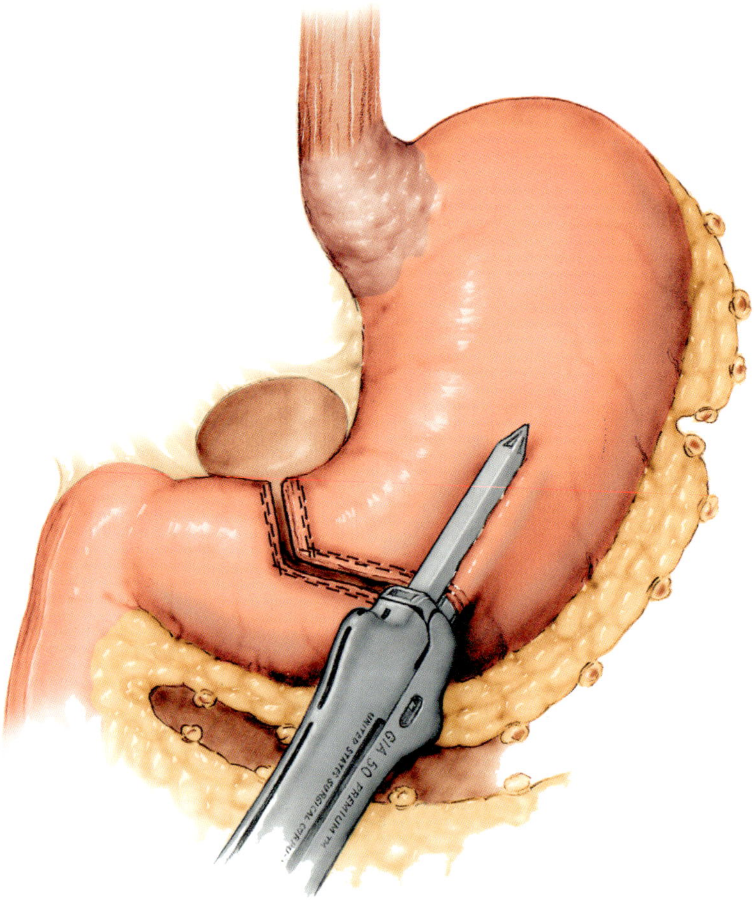

Figure III-16,B: The proximal gastric resection and distal isoperistaltic tube construction are performed by serial applications of the GIA instrument as delineated in Figure III-16,A. A Kocher maneuver is performed to increase mobility of the tube in reaching the esophagus without tension.

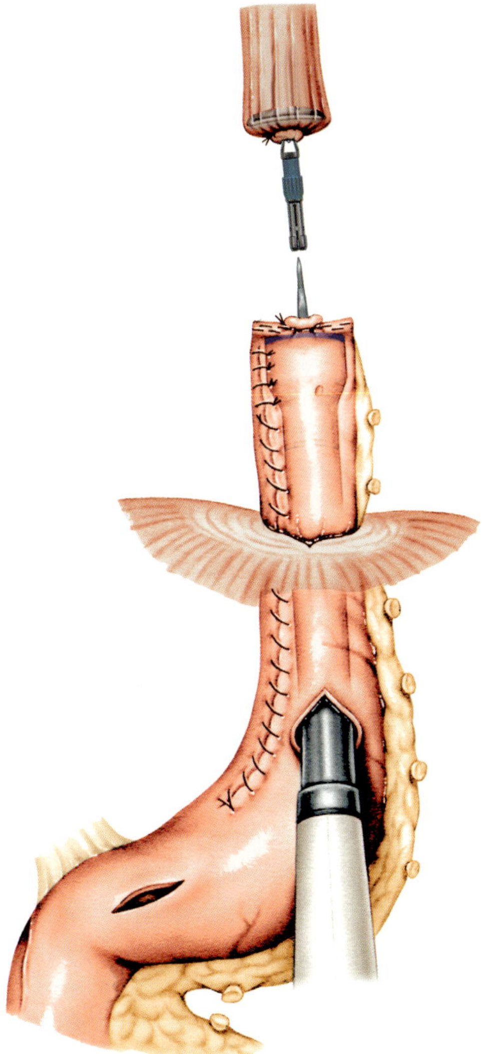

Figure III-16,C: The gastric tube staple line is reinforced with inverting interrupted sutures or a continuous running suture; however, the sutures at the projected anastomotic site should be interrupted if a running suture has been used. The esophagus is transected proximally and the specimen is removed. The open esophageal stump is prepared with a 2-0, monofilament, over-and-over whipstitch as in Figure III-12,I. The anvil of the appropriate size EEA instrument is inserted into the proximal esophagus and the purse-string suture tied securely. (A Purstring instrument can be used as in Figure III-5, A to D or the esophagus prepared as in Figure III-5, H to J for triple stapling technique). The EEA instrument, without anvil, is introduced through a low gastrotomy and advanced to the stapled proximal end of the tube. A small incision at the midpoint of the staple line aids in the passage of the center rod as the instrument is opened.

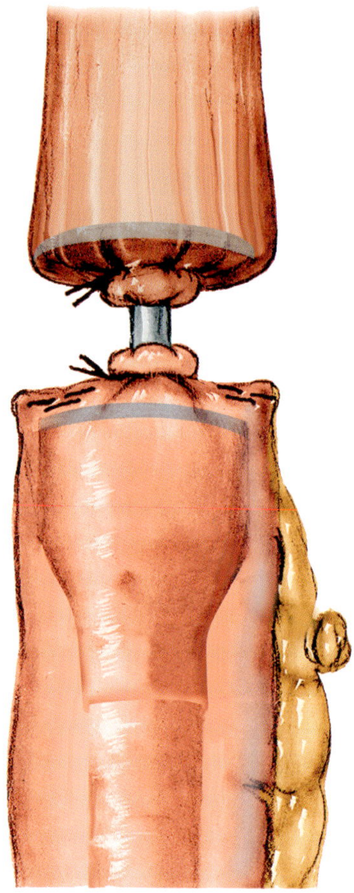

Figure III-16,D: The anvil shaft and center rod are mated and the anvil is closed against the cartridge, while care is taken to maintain all tissues snug against the cartridge and anvil to reduce the possibility of bunching or pleating of tissue participating in the anastomosis and to eliminate extraneous tissue from being incorporated between the closing anvil and cartridge.

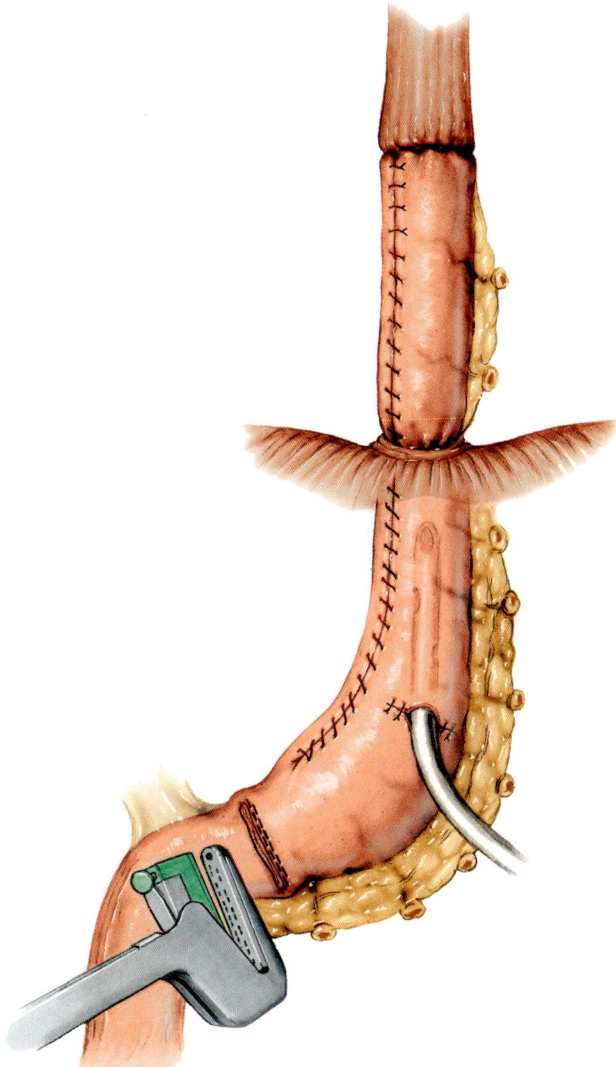

Figure III-16,E: The instrument is activated performing the transhiatal, intrathoracic, double stapling technique, end-to-end esophagogastrostomy. Following removal of the instrument, the anastomosis is examined for hemostasis prior to closure of the gastrotomy. A drainage-feeding gastrostomy is always part of any operation where a remnant of stomach remains below the diaphragm. The gastrostomy tube is placed through the gastrotomy and the remainder of the incision is closed around it. Pyloroplasty or pyloromyotomy are optional. The slender gastric tube forms a smooth transition with the normal caliber of the proximal esophagus.

Alternatively, the technique shown in Figure III-15, A to C may be used.

ESOPHAGOGASTRECTOMY AND COLON INTERPOSITION

Distal esophagectomy, proximal gastrectomy, and replacement with a transverse colon segment can be performed for malignant disease in case of a previous subtotal gastrectomy or for benign fibrous strictures due to gastroesophageal reflux or caustic burns.

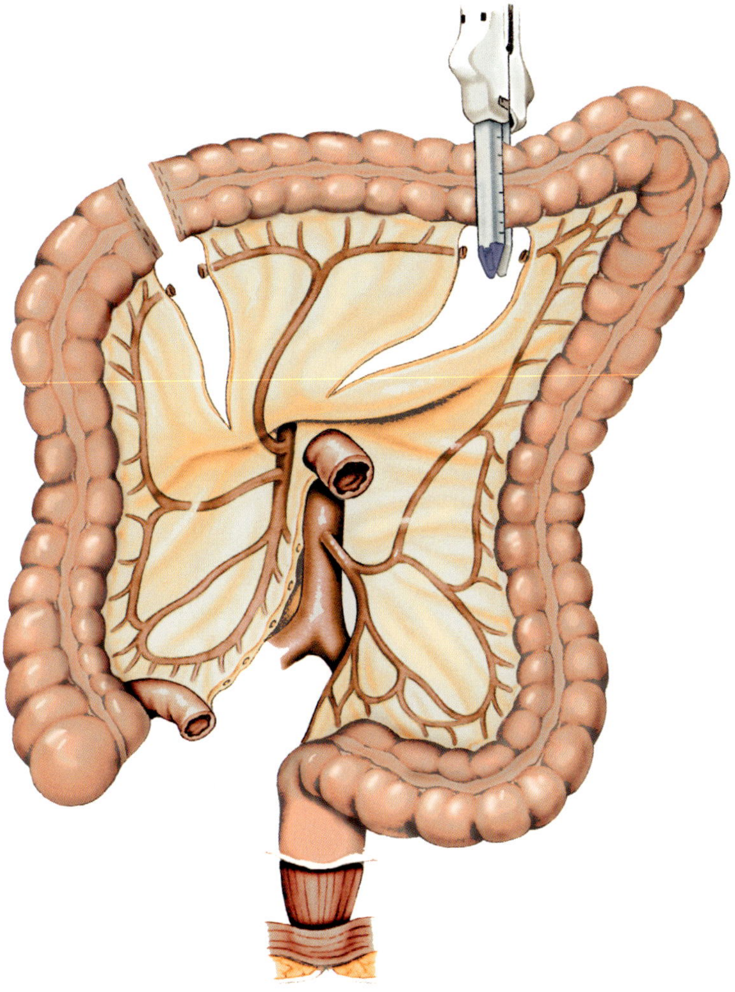

Figure III-17,A: The segment of colon required depends on the extent of the gap to be bridged and may be much shorter, at other times longer, than that shown here. It may be used in an isoperistaltic or antiperistaltic fashion, depending on the mobility of the middle colic vessels and the configuration of their right and left branches. The marginal vessels to and from the segment of transverse colon chosen are ligated and divided at the points of proximal and distal colon transection, and established at a distance from each other that provides the desired length of bowel for the replacement. The GIA instrument is used to close and transect the colon proximally and distally.

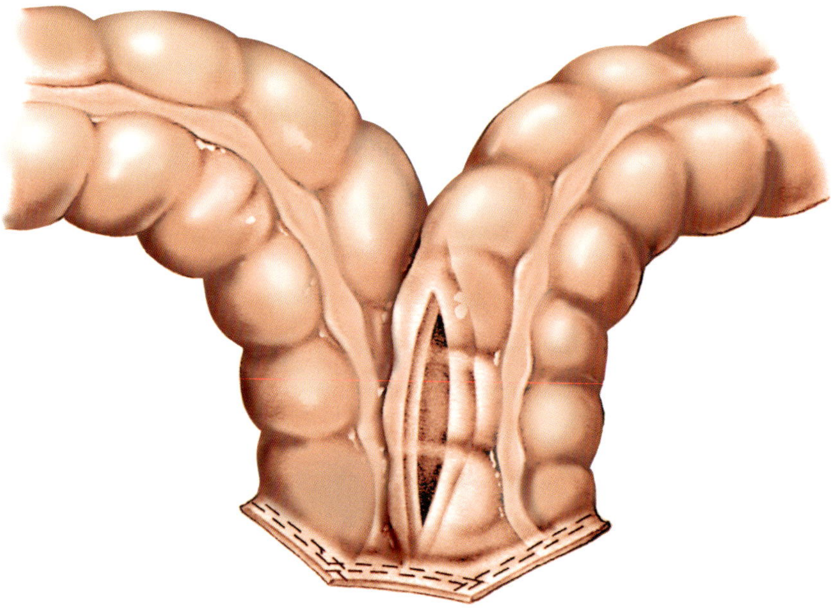

Figure III-17,B: The colocolostomy to re-establish intestinal continuity is performed in a functional end-to-end fashion (similar to the ileocolostomy described in Figure III-8, G to I).

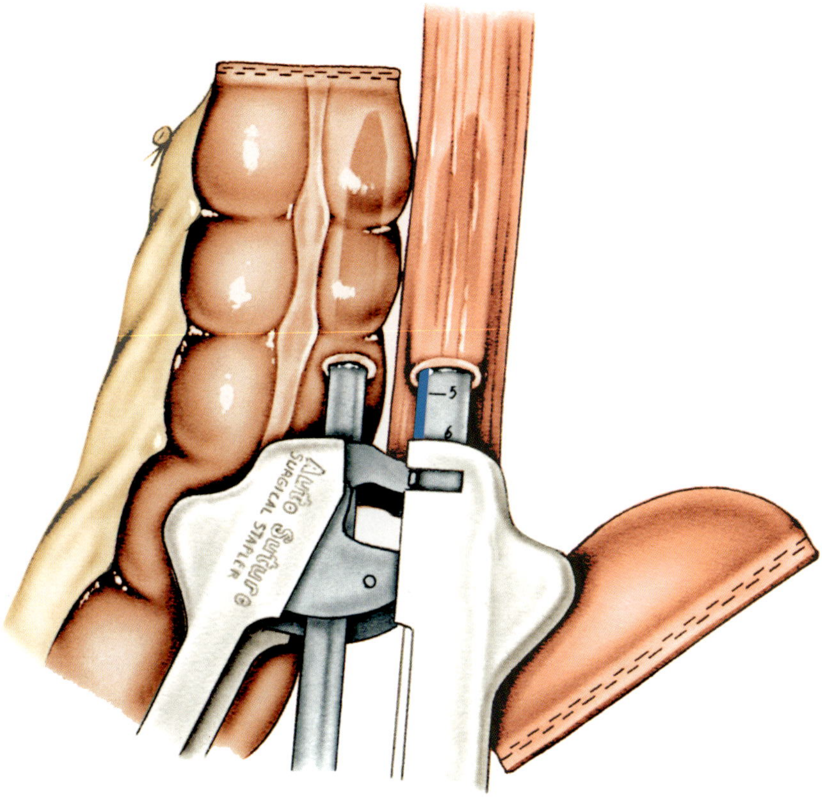

Figure III-17,C: The gastric fundus is closed with two parallel TA 90 staple lines and divided between these transverse, parallel staple closures as in Figure III-12, A and B. The esophagus is freed into the mediastinum by using the cardia as a convenient handle, and the colon is brought up behind the stomach into the posterior mediastinum alongside the esophagus. If the segment of colon needed to span the defect is long, a side-to-side esophagocolostomy with the linear anastomosing instrument is preferable since it provides greater versatility in adjusting convenience of instrumentation to individual technical requirements.

As in the linear esophagocolic anastomosis in the neck, the GIA instrument is placed through kissing stab wounds, with one fork into the esophagus at the selected site of transection and one fork into the colon segment at a 5 to 6 cm distance from its closed proximal end (Figure III-8,N). The instrument halves are mated, the instrument is closed and activated, and the side-to-side anastomosis is performed, while using the esophagogastric specimen as a convenient handle.

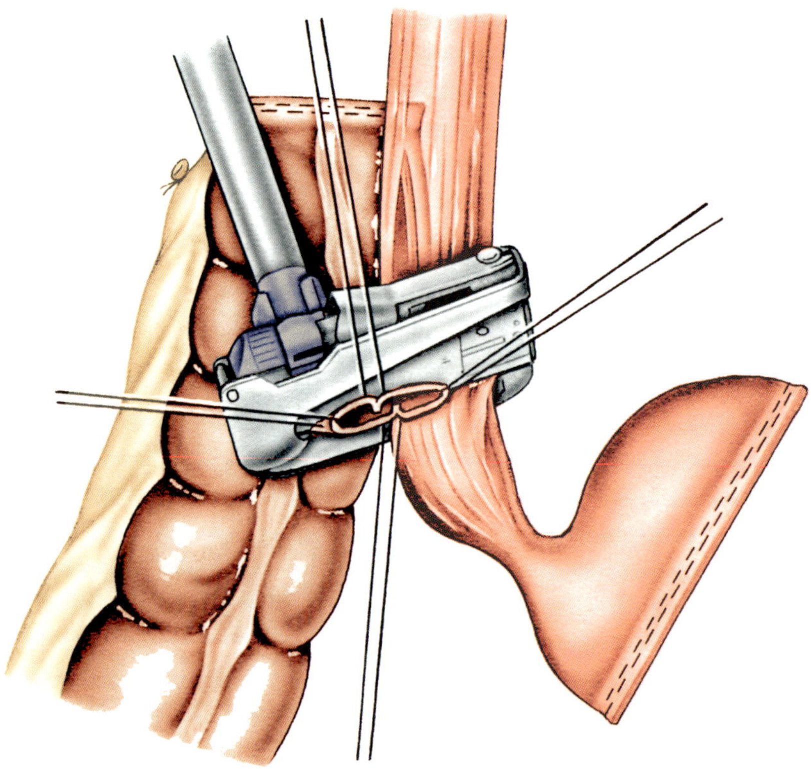

Figure III-17,D: After removal of the GIA instrument and inspection of the anastomosis for hemostasis, the oblique placement of the TA instrument (as in Figure III-8,O), across the now common GIA introduction site and the remaining circumference of the esophagus proximal to this site, permits the simultaneous stapling of the esophagus and the common GIA opening.

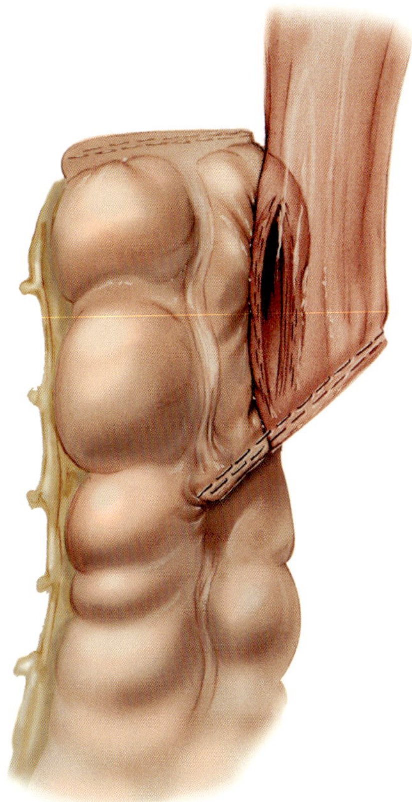

Figure III-17,E: Resection of the specimen ("anastomose-resection integree"), using the caudad edge of the TA instrument as a guide, completes this type of anastomosis.

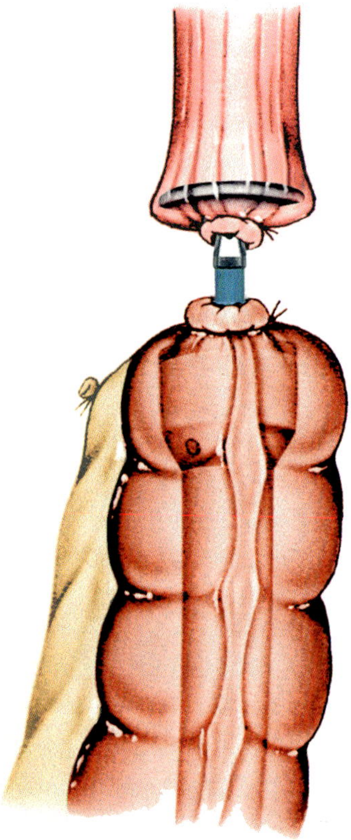

Figure III-17,F: If the segment of interposed colon is short, allowing for the comfortable use of the circular stapling instrument to bridge the defect, the EEA can be placed through the opened distal end of the colon substitute and carried into the lower mediastinum. A classical end-to-end esophagocolostomy is then performed with the circular anastomosing instrument, similar to that shown in Fiqure III-8, P and Q.

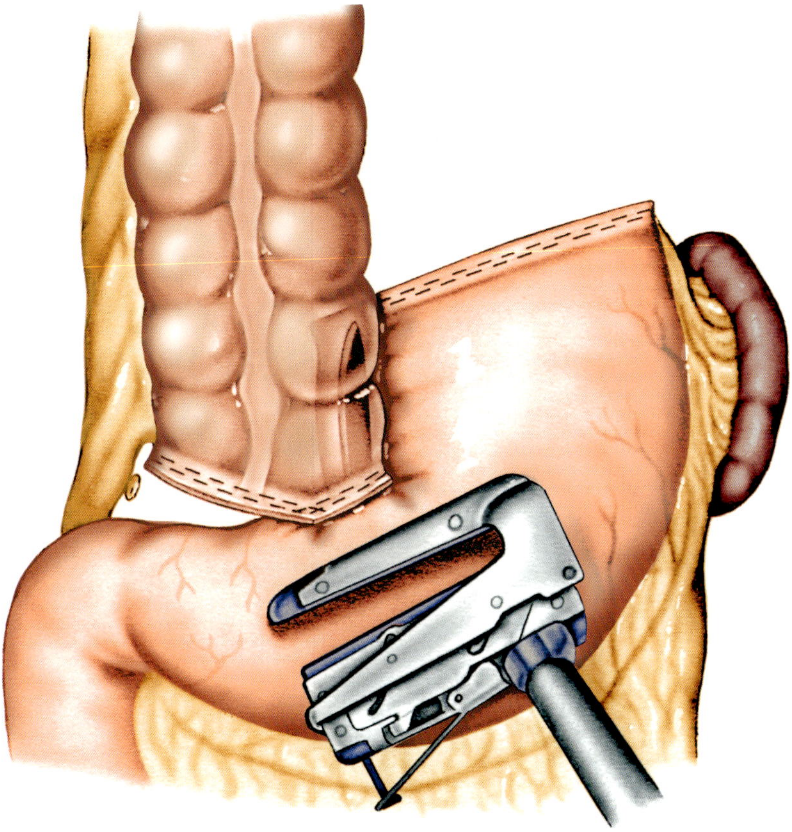

Figure III-17,G: To re-establish distal continuity, the segment of colon is tailored to the exact length required— if necessary—and closed once more with a transverse TA staple line, regardless of the type of proximal anastomosis (i.e., end-to-end or side-to-side). A side-to-side cologastrostomy is performed with the GIA instrument forks inserted into the colon through its excised antimesocolic corner and into the gastric remnant through a stab wound into the anterior wall of the stomach along the lesser curvature. After accomplishing the side-to-side anastomosis and removing the GIA instrument, the common stab wound opening is closed with a linear stapler.

PALLIATIVE END-TO-SIDE ESOPHAGOGASTROSTOMY

Palliative bypass esophagogastrostomy is performed for inoperable lower third or GE junction carcinoma in patients who can be expected to have a near-normal grace period, possibly enhanced with radiotherapy and/or chemotherapy. Nutrition by open upper esophagogastric passages and the elimination of tracheobronchial aspiration due to complete esophageal obstruction can greatly improve the temporary quality of life for such patients.

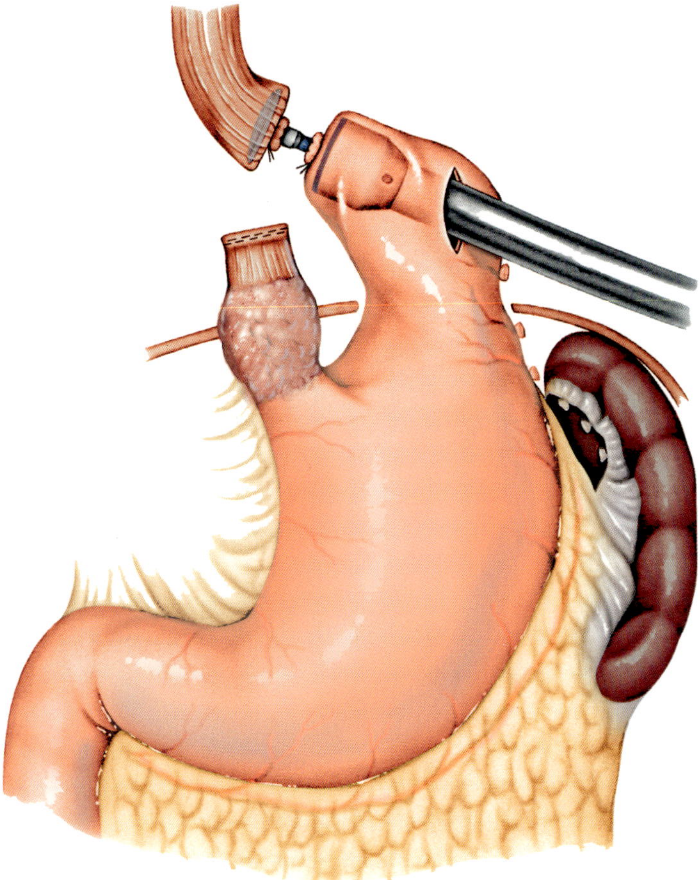

Figure III-18,A: Through a left thoracic approach, the lower esophagus is dissected and stapled transversely above the tumor. The fundus and greater gastric curvature are liberated through an incision in the tendinous portion of the diaphragm. Several short gastric vessels are tied and transected. The anvil is placed into the proximal esophagus and secured with the usual purse-string suture. The cartridge-bearing EEA instrument is advanced through a gastrotomy into the fundus that has been rolled into the chest through a phrenotomy in the tendinous portion of the diaphragm. End-to-side anastomosis is performed entirely through the chest incision, and the diaphragm is loosely closed around the stomach.

PALLIATIVE SIDE-TO-SIDE ESOPHAGOGASTROSTOMY

The palliative bypass, first described by Martin Kirschner of Konigsberg (then Germany, now Poland) in 1920 and "reactivated" by Paul Kirschner (no relation) of Mount Sinai Hospital in New York in the 1980s, can also be performed with the linear anastomosing instrument.

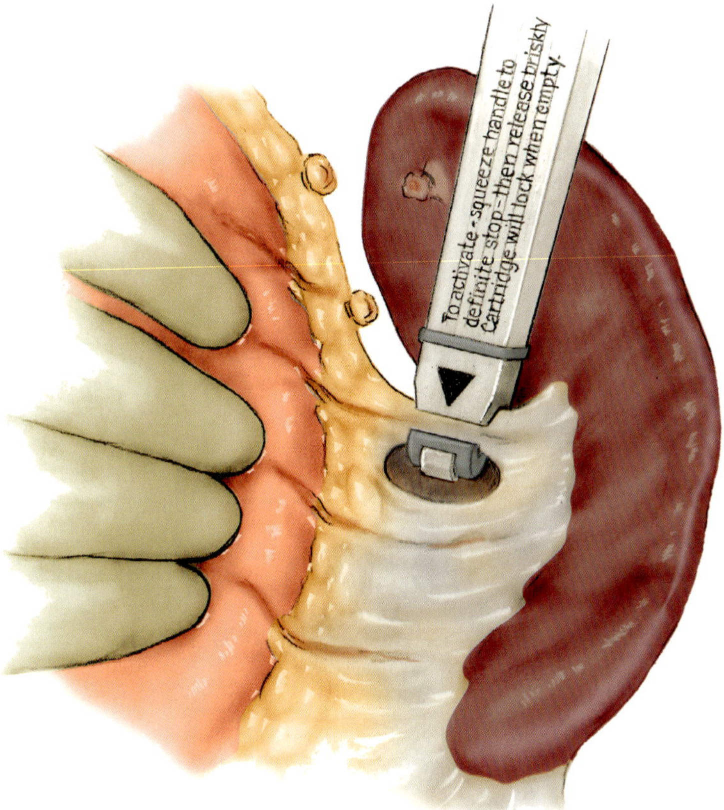

Figure III-19,A: The LDS instrument is used to mobilize the fundus of the stomach by ligating and dividing the first three or four vasa brevia, leaving the spleen intact.

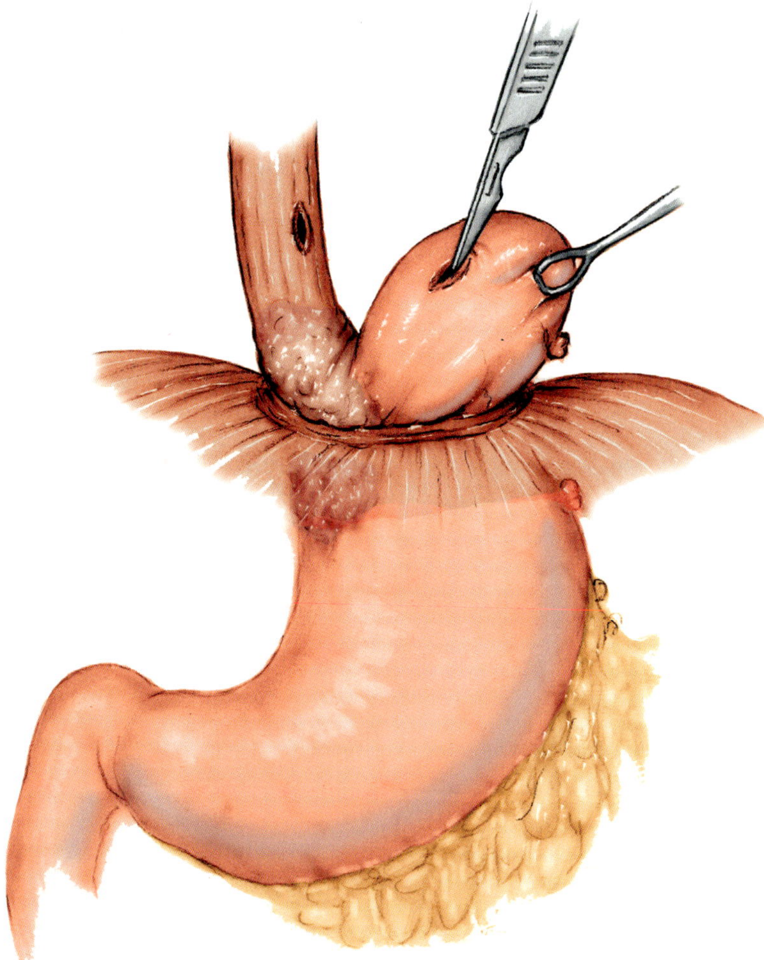

Figure III-19,B: The fundus is elevated into the lower mediastinum through an enlarged diaphragmatic hiatus and positioned alongside the esophagus. Parallel stab wounds are made into the lateral wall of the esophagus, 5 to 6 cm proximal to the tumor and the medial wall of the fundus.

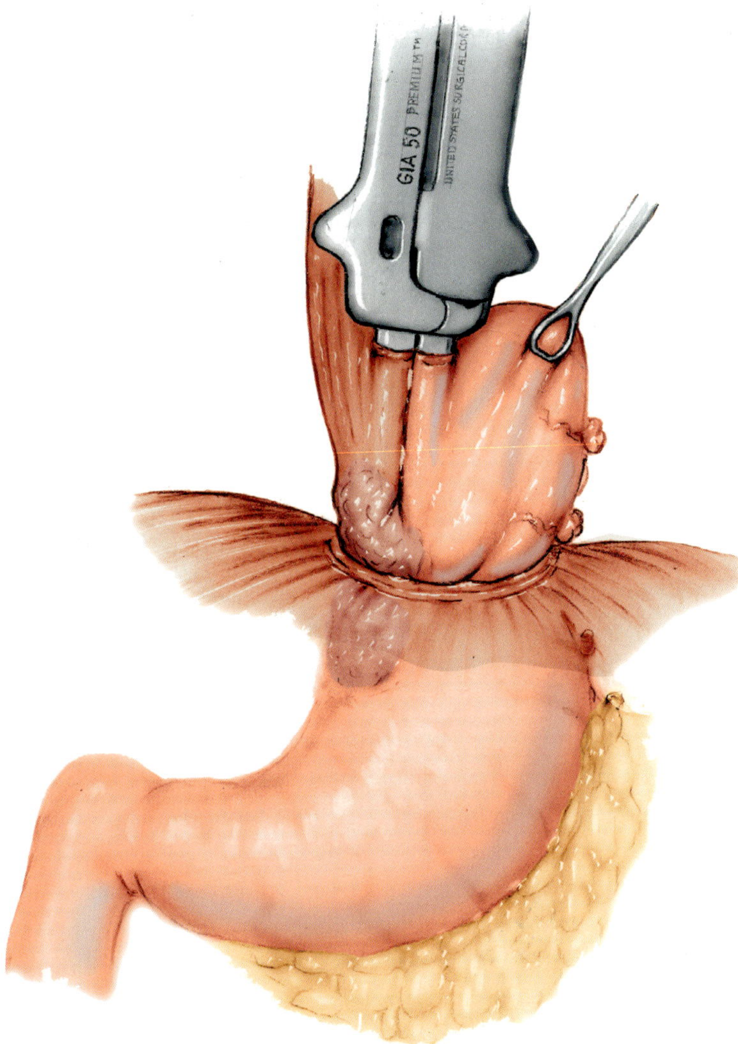

Figure III-19,C: One fork of the GIA instrument is placed into each lumen and advanced caudally. The instrument halves are joined, the tissue is evenly aligned on the forks, and the instrument is closed and activated. The anastomosis is inspected for hemostasis prior to closure of the common opening with a linear stapler or manual sutures.

THORACIC COLLIS-NISSEN PROCEDURE

Collis gastroplasty and Nissen fundoplication are indicated for soft, dilatable esophageal strictures associated with a shortened esophagus, firmly attached to the surrounding mediastinum by tough fibrous, post-inflammatory adhesions. The shortening of the esophagus is due to retraction of the abdominal esophagus into the mediastinum, and the entire clinical picture is the consequence of esophageal reflux, esophagitis, and periesophagitis. Rather than risking a difficult dissection and permanent severance of scarce blood supply to bring the scarred lower esophagus below the diaphragm, or worse, gambling on the antireflux effect of a fundoplication above the diaphragm in the face of a high incidence of inherent complications (ulceration, bleeding, perforation, gastro-pericardial fistula), it is preferable to elongate the esophagus by a Collis gastroplasty. A ring of gastric fundus can then encircle the new intra-abdominal neoesophagus to prevent further reflux. However, this entire therapeutic scenario is only possible if the esophageal stricture is dilatable preoperatively and intraoperatively. If this is not the case, a colon interposition must be used to overcome dysphagia and bronchopulmonary aspiration due to stricture, as well as to eliminate the threat of malignant transformation of chronic esophagitis and still prevent further reflux through the mechanical barrier of an acid-resistant segment of colon. In the occasional marginal case, the patient and the surgeon have to be prepared to switch intraoperatively from a planned Collis-Nissen procedure to a contingency oriented colon interposition.

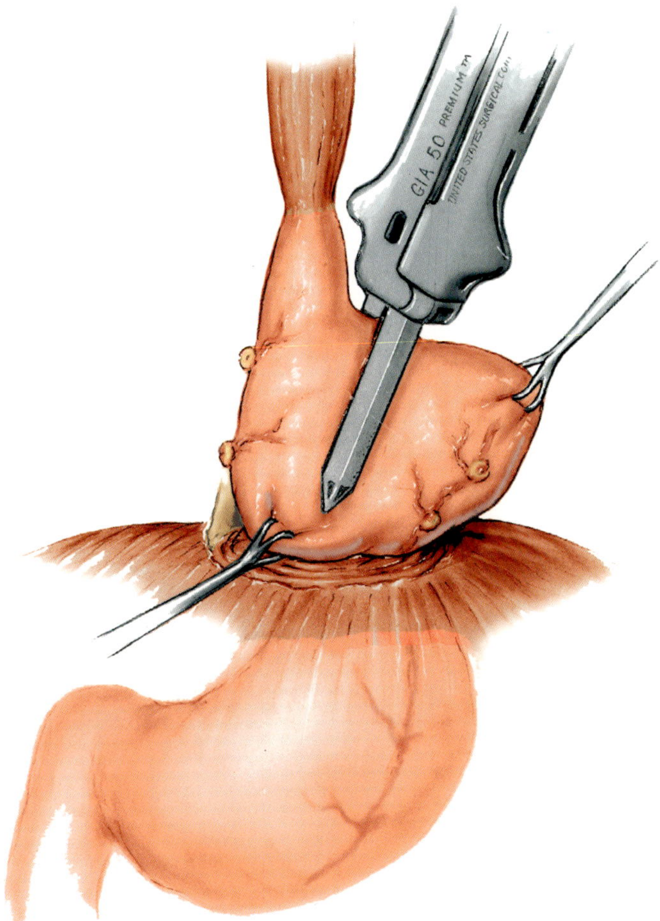

Figure III-20,A: With shortening and retraction of the abdominal esophagus into the mediastinum due to esophagitis, the GE junction is pulled up through the enlarged hiatus, as a sliding hiatal hernia. It is a simple matter to enlarge the hiatus and mobilize additional gastric fundus in order to accommodate the GIA instrument in creating a 5 to 6 cm gastric tube in continuity with the esophagus. The lumen of the neoesophagus is calibrated with an indwelling large bougie.

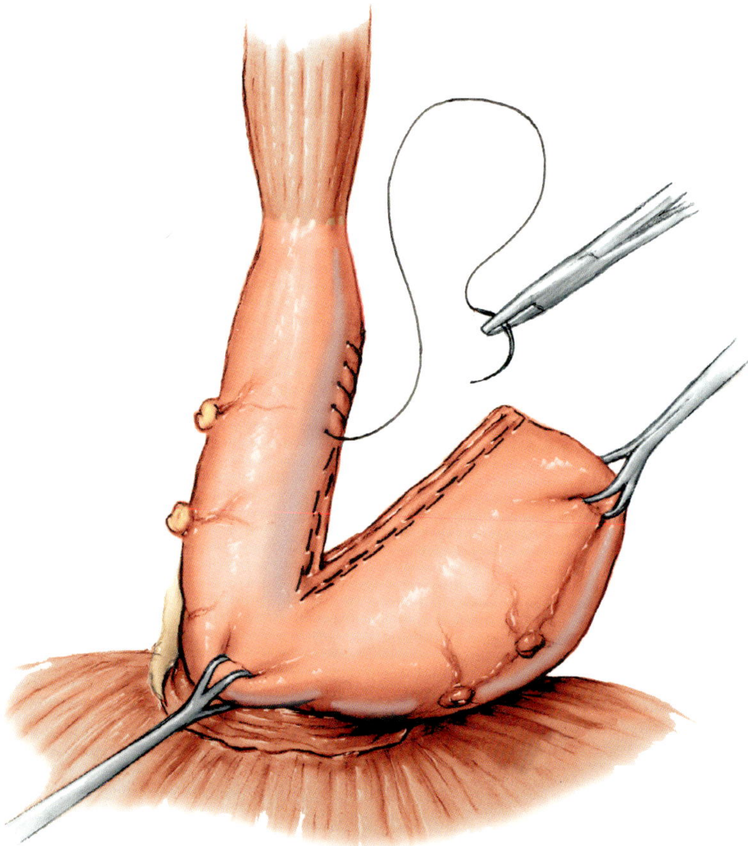

Figure III-20,B: As in all applications of the GIA instrument on a double thickness of gastric wall, the GIA staple lines are reinforced with a running suture.

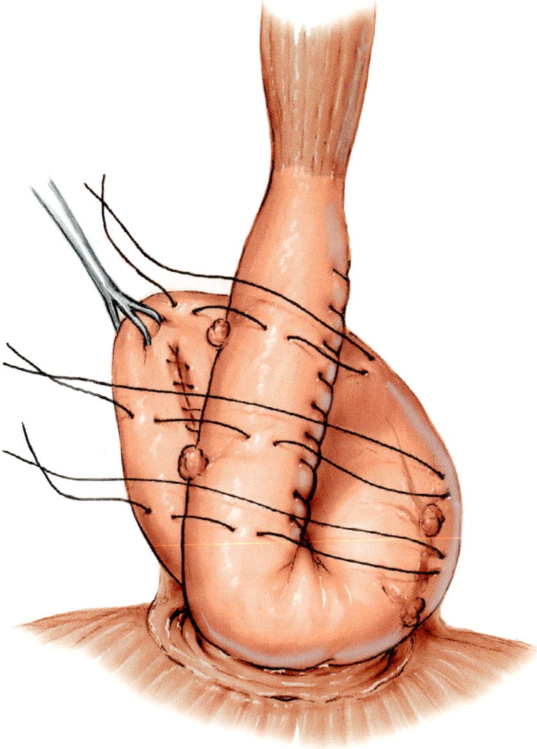

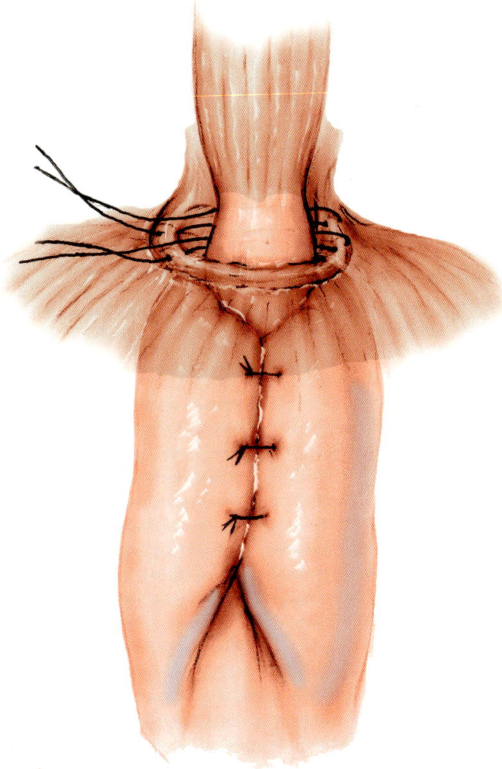

Figure III-20,C: A Nissen wrap is performed by swinging the flap of fundus obtained by the GIA transection around the neoesophagus and suturing its tip to the body of the stomach on the left side of the "new" esophagus.

Figure III-20,D: The stomach is replaced below the diaphragm and the hiatus closed around the tubed portion of the stomach, just distal to the stricture.

ABDOMINAL COLLIS-NISSEN PROCEDURE

In the elderly patient with poor cardiac reserve and pulmonary restrictions due to repeated episodes of aspiration, thoracotomy is not as well tolerated as is laparotomy. The technique of a Collis gastroplasty-Nissen fundoplication can be safely performed through an abdominal approach if the GE junction is located within the lower third of the mediastinum, making a transhiatal dissection of the sliding cardia and placement of the GIA tips into the mediatinum possible.

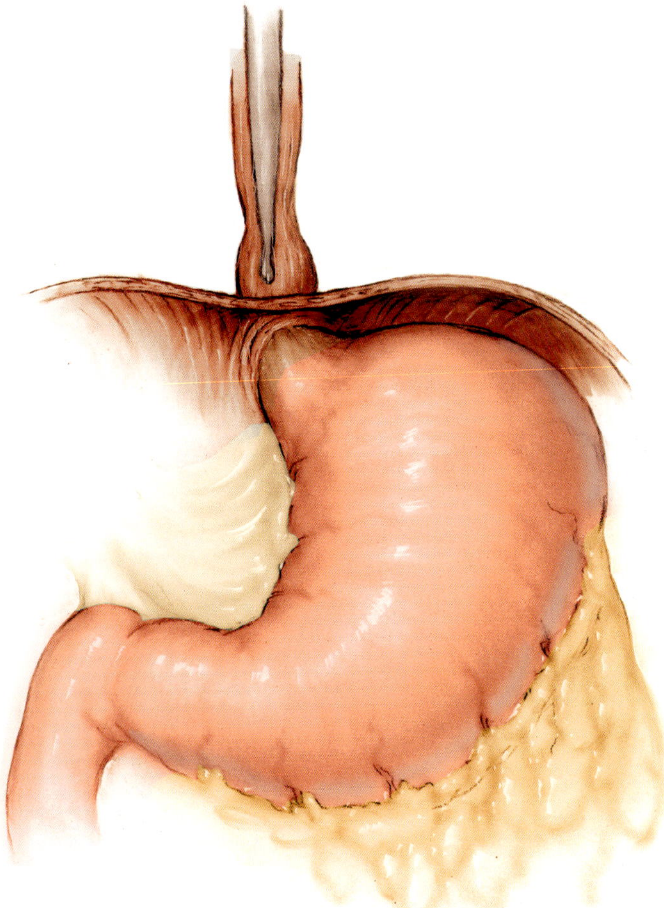

Figure III-21,A: A French #50-52 bougie is introduced to dilate the stricture and to act as a guide for the creation of the gastric tube.

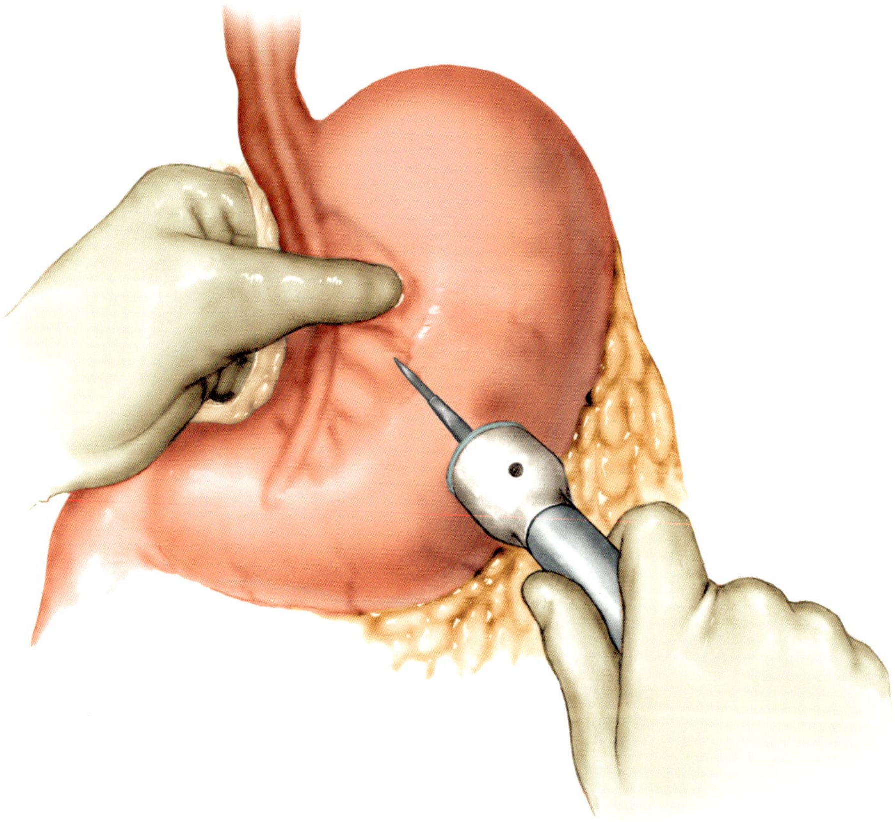

Figure III-21,B: To facilitate the placement of the GIA instrument on the stomach for the creation of the gastric tube in prolongation of the esophagus, a buttonhole is created with the EEA 21 instrument about 5 cm below the angle of His and inside the lesser curvature, at a distance equal to the width of the esophagus. An opening is made in the avascular space of the lesser omentum for access of the surgeon's left index finger to fifth finger behind the posterior wall of the stomach. The EEA instrument, without anvil, is prepared by advancing the center rod so that the tip will perforate both gastric walls at the center of the placement selected for the buttonhole, while the lesser curvature is held in position between the left thumb and the long fingers.

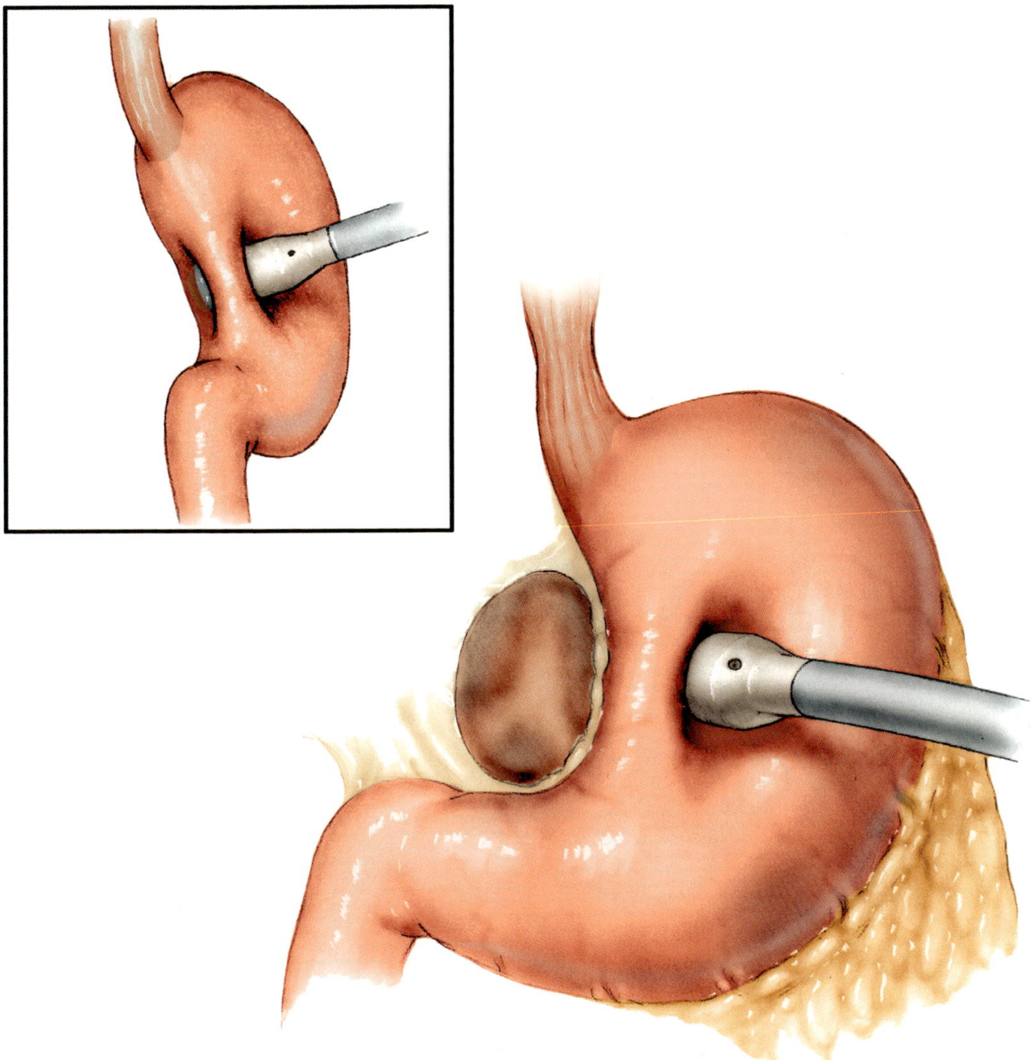

Figure III-21,C,D: After penetrating through both walls of the stomach, the anvil is transported posteriorly and mated with the center rod of the EEA instrument. The instrument is closed, compressing the anterior and posterior walls of the stomach, and is activated, placing a circular double staggered staple line joining the gastric walls and cutting out a buttonhole.

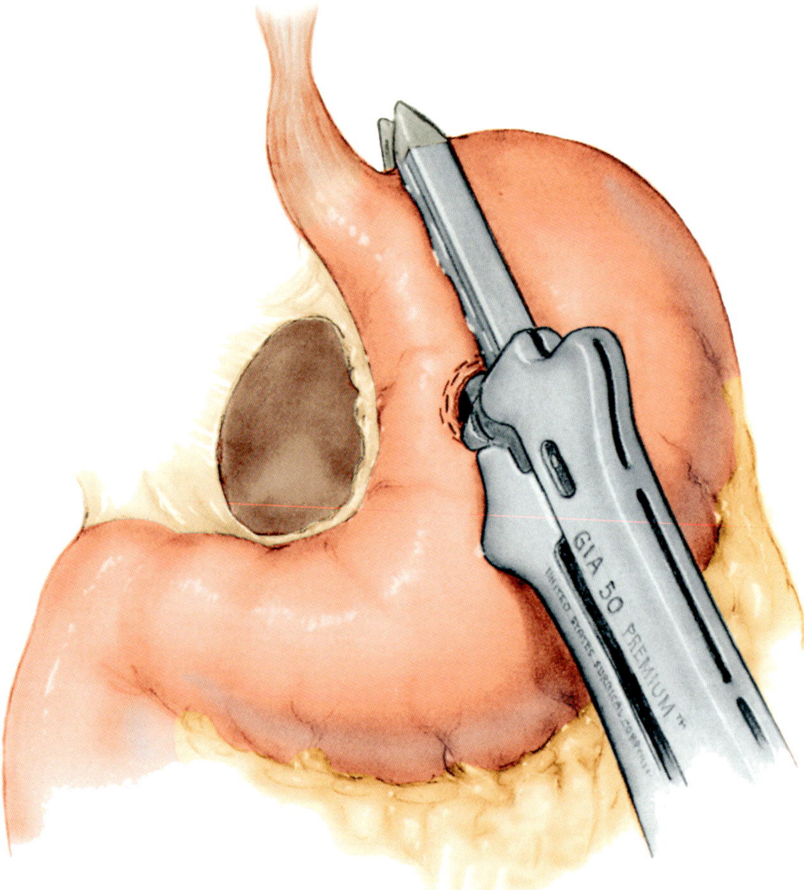

Figure III-21,E: The GIA instrument is placed parallel to and inside the lesser curvature, with one fork inside the lesser sac and one fork on the anterior wall of the stomach. The instrument is activated and the Collis gastroplasty created.

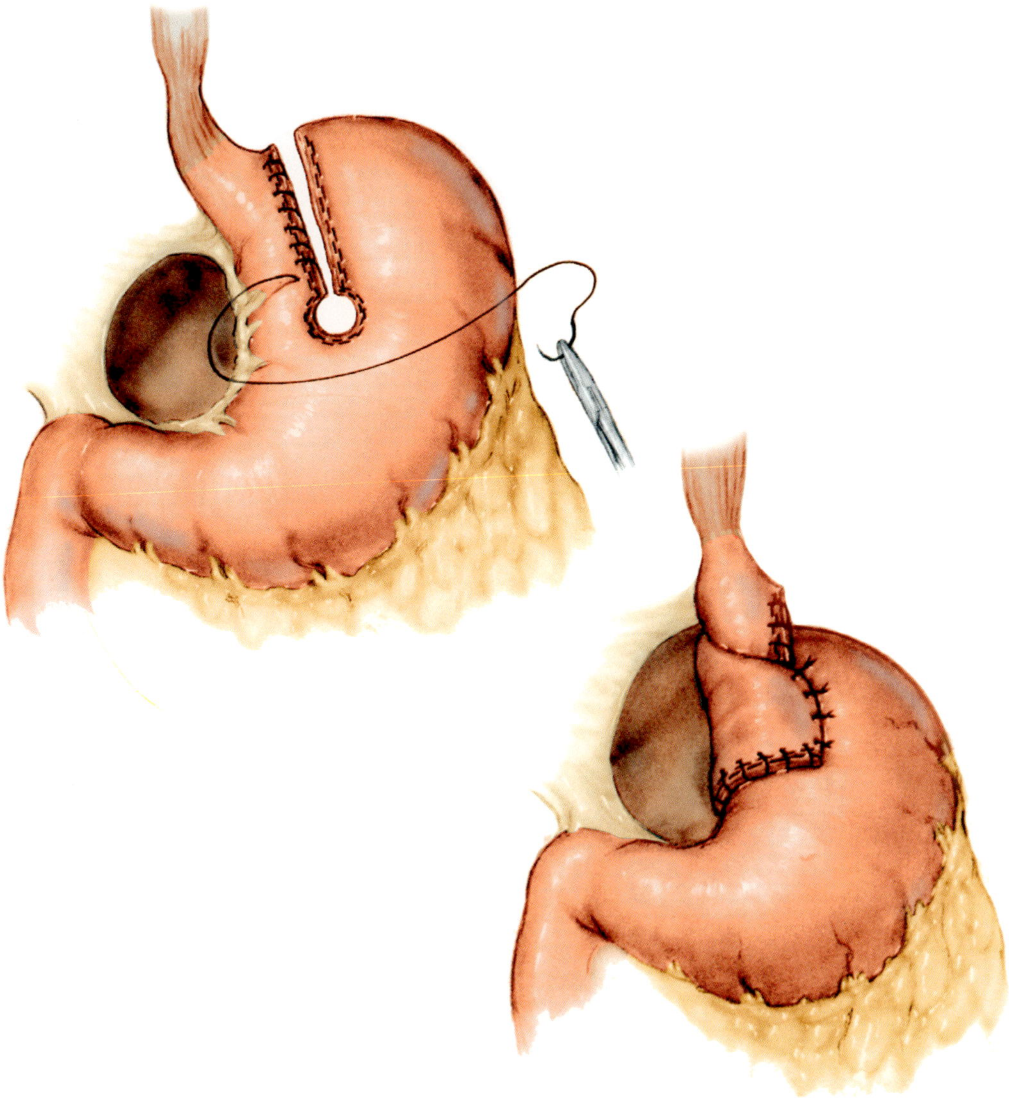

Figure III-21,F: As for all applications of the GIA instrument on a double thickness of gastric wall, the GIA staple lines are reinforced with running sutures.

Figure III-21,G: The remaining "neofundus," or dog ear, is swung posteriorly around the tubed gastric prolongation of the esophagus. The tip of the dog ear is sutured anteriorly to its base and the modified Nissen fundoplication completed.

LIGATION OF ESOPHAGEAL VARICES

This procedure is part of the porto-azygos disconnection operation developed by Del Guercio for the treatment of acute variceal bleeding. It has become somewhat of a historical standby in the age of the transjugular intrahepatic portosystemic shunt (TIPS) procedure, for institutions that do not treat variceal bleeding with any regularity, but may have to take care of the occasional patient who can not be transferred safely to a center with TIPS expertise. The ligation can be performed with the EEA or GIA instruments.

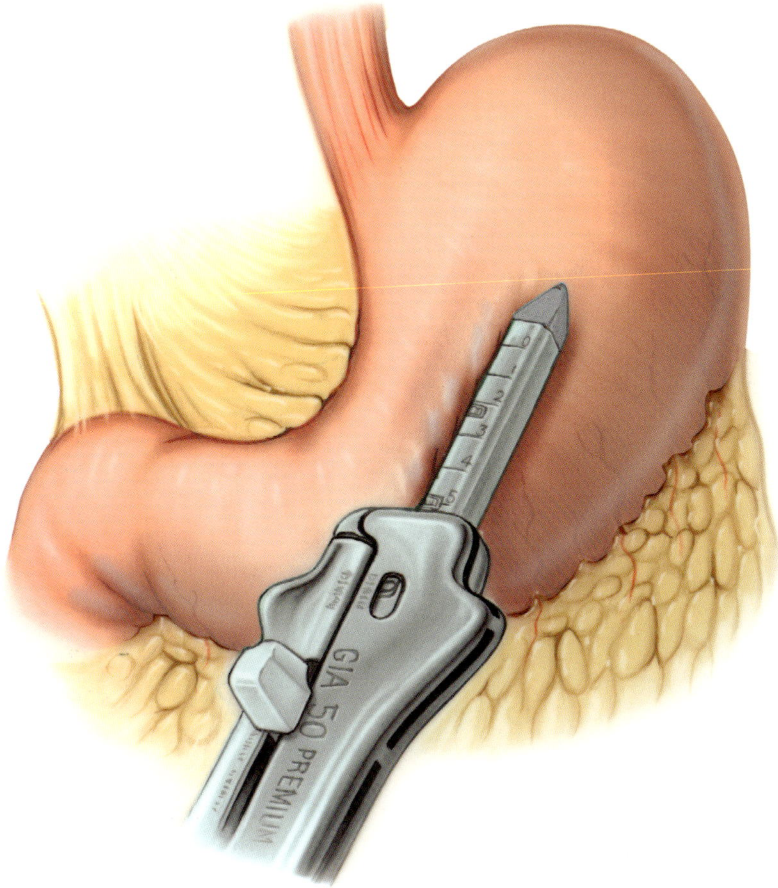

Figure III-22,A: For the EEA-guided procedure, the GIA instrument is used to create an anterior gastrotomy. A 1 cm stab wound is made into the midanterior gastric wall. The anvil fork of the GIA instrument is inserted into the lumen of the stomach and advanced cephalad to the distance required for an opening to accommodate the appropriate size EEA instrument. The cartridge fork is placed on the serosal surface, and the instrument is closed, activated, and removed.

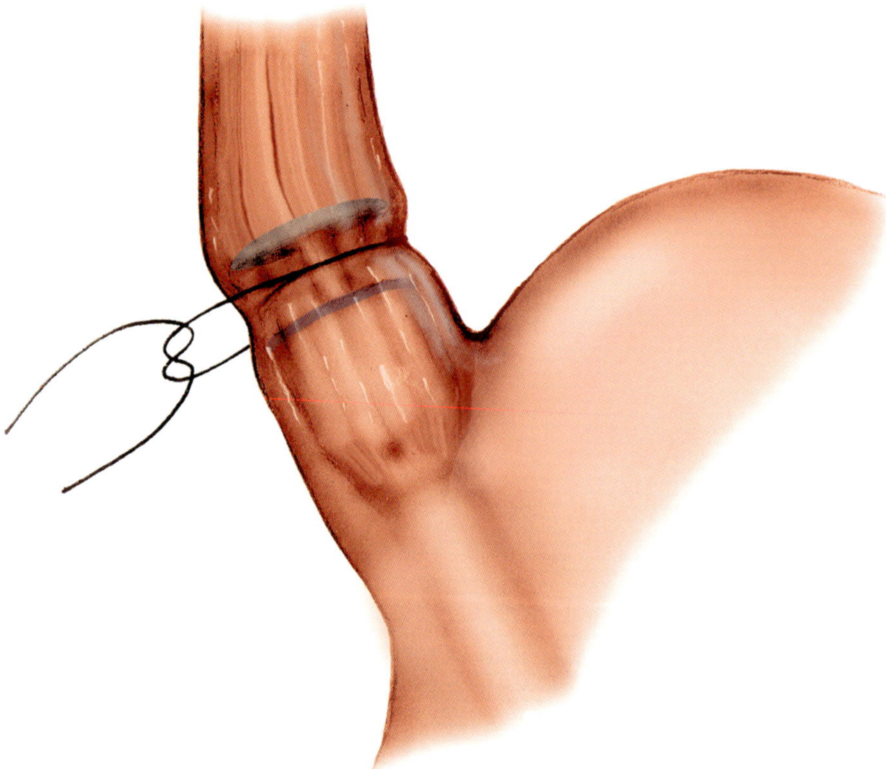

Figure III-22,B: The EEA instrument is introduced through the gastrotomy and advanced into the distal esophagus. The instrument is opened, separating the anvil from the cartridge, and a ligature is tied around the esophagus, between the anvil and cartridge, down to the center rod of the instrument.

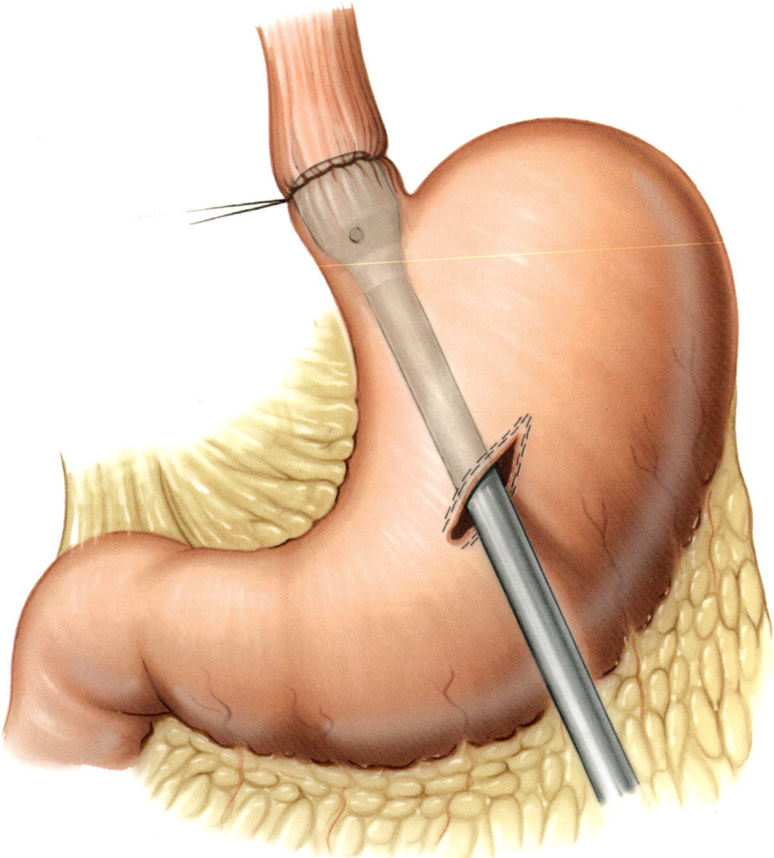

Figure III-22,C: The instrument is closed—anvil against cartridge, taking care that no extraneous tissue is incorporated—and activated.

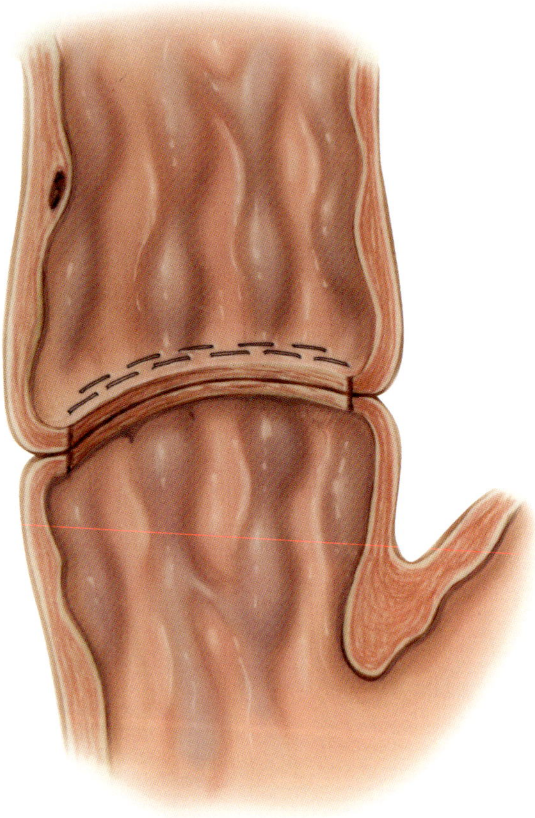

Figure III-22,D: The EEA instrument places a circular, double staggered row of staples that ligates the esophageal varices, and the knife blade cuts a stoma.

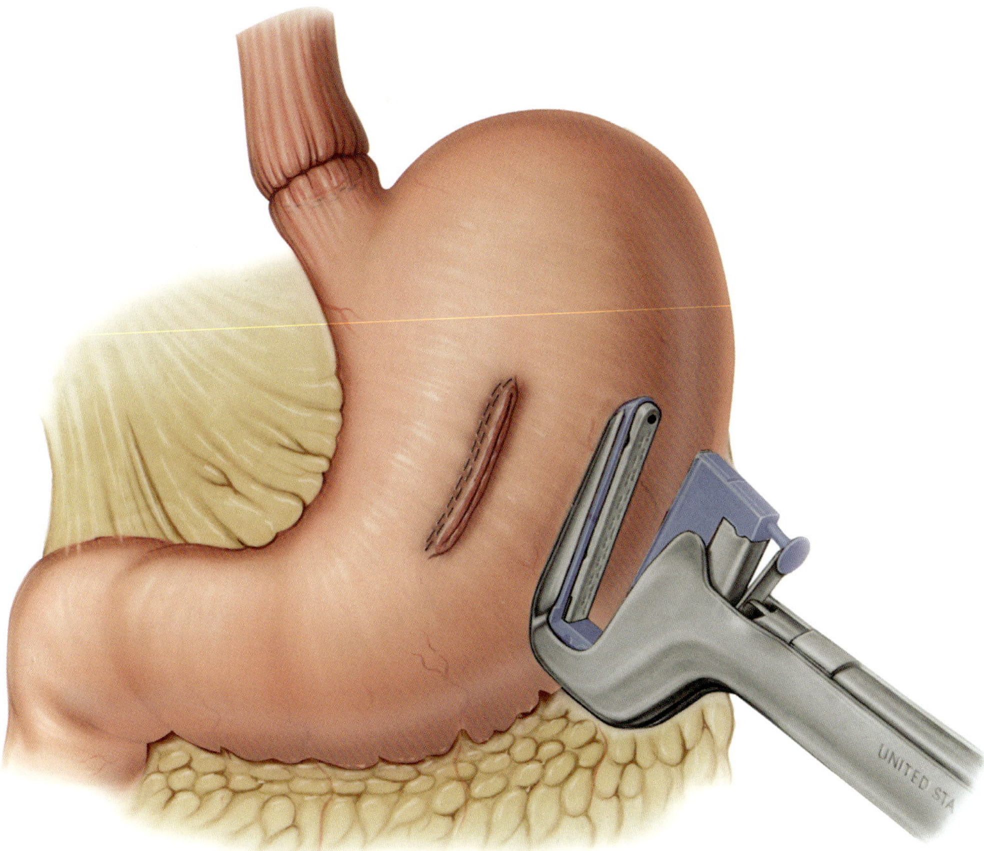

Figure III-22,E: The instrument is opened and removed, and the stoma inspected for hemostasis prior to closure of the gastrotomy with a linear stapler.

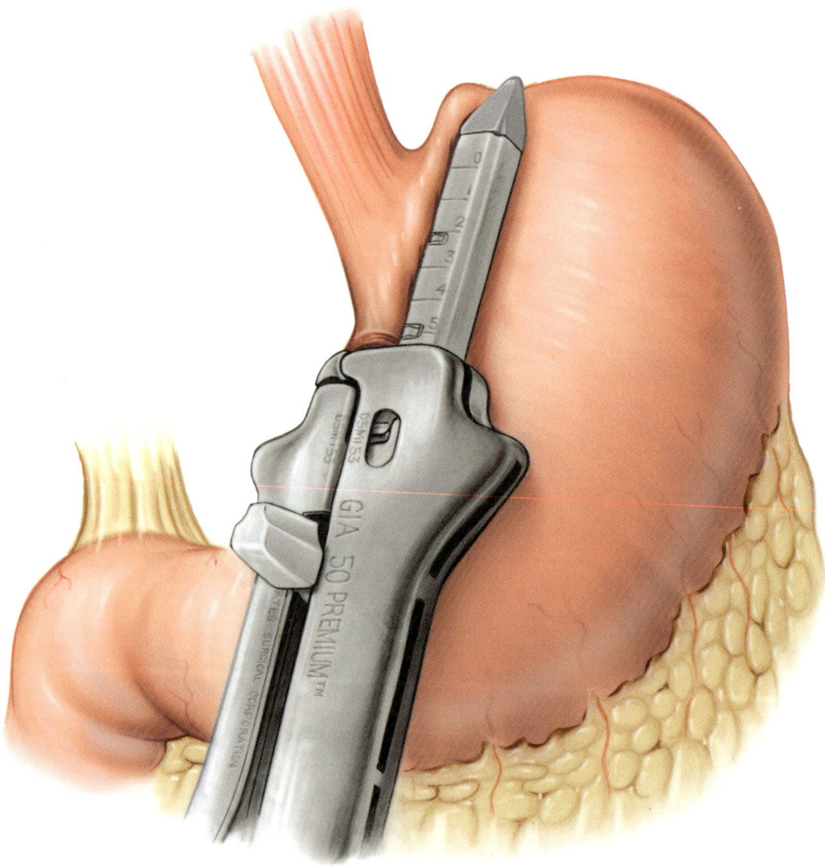

Figure III-22,F: Alternatively, the varices can be ligated distal to the esophagogastric junction using the GIA instrument loaded with a cartridge that contains no knife blade, as first proposed by Rinecker and Danek from Munich in 1975. A 1 cm stab wound is made into the lesser curvature of the stomach just distal to the junction. The anvil fork of the instrument is inserted into the lumen of the stomach and the cartridge fork placed on the anterior serosal surface. The instrument is closed, activated, and removed.

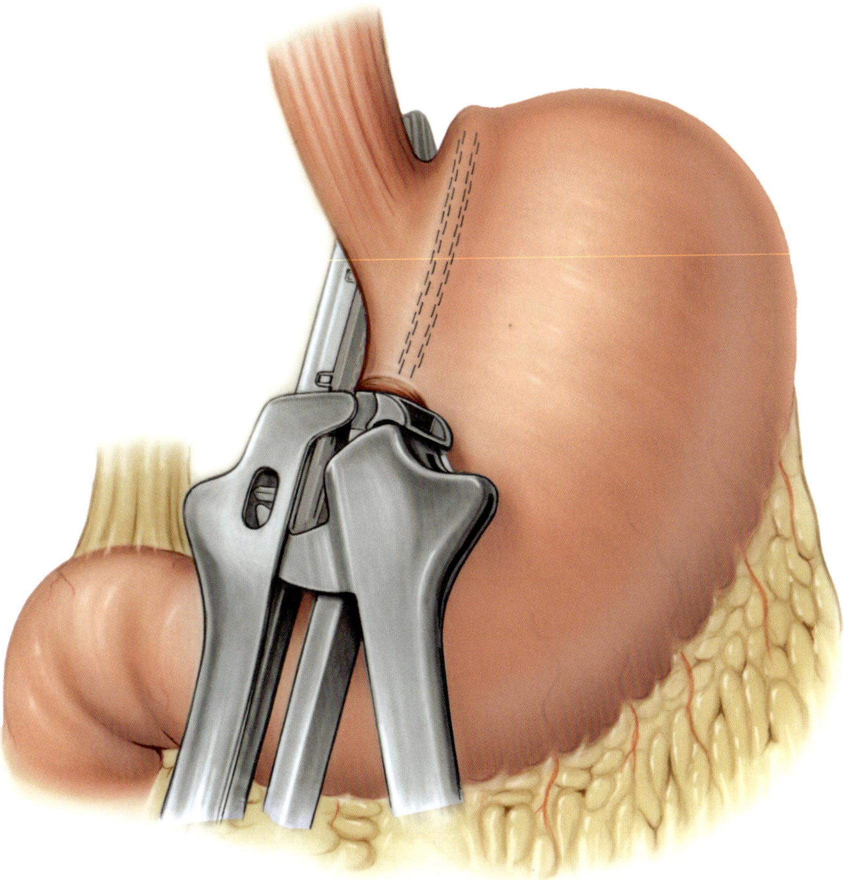

Figure III-22,G: The instrument is reloaded and reapplied similarly on the posterior wall of the stomach. The staple lines are inspected, and the stab wound is closed with the TA 30 instrument or manual sutures.

TABLE III-1
Evaluation of Stapled Esophagogastric Anastomoses in Literature

Author	Instrument	No. of Cases	Leak	Resulting Mortality
Behl et al	EEA	40	1 (2.5%)	1 (2.5%)
Dickson	EEA & ILS*	59	0	0
Donnelly et al	EEA	195	4 (2.1%)	1 (0.5%)
Dorsey et al	EEA	9	0	0
Fekete et al	EEA	127	7 (5.5%)	0
	ILS*	73	3 (4.1%)	0
Hopkins et al	EEA	60	1 (1.7%)	0
Imaniura et al	EEA	10	0	0
Kaplan et al	EEA	164	3 (1.8%)	1 (0.6%)
Kivelitz & Ulrich	EEA	19	0	0
Kockel & Ulrich	EEA	35	3 (8.6%)	1 (2.9%)
Page et al	EEA	115	2 (1.7%)	1 (0.9%)
Shahinian et al	EEA	10	0	0
Spina et al	EEA	17	1 (5.9%)	0
Sugimachi et al	EEA	11	0	0
	SPTU	17	1 (5.9%)	?
West et al	EEA	31	0	0
Wilson et al	EEA	30	1 (3.3%)	0
Wong et al	EEA & ILS*	146	5 (3.5%)	0
Woods et al	EEA	49	0	0
	ILS*	1	0	0
Totals		**1218**	**32 (2.6%)**	**5 (0.4%)**

Table III-2
Occurrence of Benign Esophageal Strictures in Literature

Author	Instrument	No. of Cases	No. of Strictures
Dickson	EEA & ILS*	59	3 (5.0%)
Donnelly et al	EEA	95	22 (13.1%)
Imamura et al	EEA	10	0
Kaplan et al	EEA	64	16 (9.7%)
Kockel & Ulrich	ILS*	11	1 (9.1%)
Page et al	EEA	15	16 (13.9%)
Wong et al	EEA & ILS*	115	16 (13.9%)
Woods et al	EEA	49	0
	ILS*	1	0
Totals		**719**	**74 (10.3%)**

In most cases, strictures were resolved by dilatation only.

* ILS is a registered trademark of Ethicon Endo-Surgery, Inc., a Johnson & Johnson Company

An update by Sugimachi published in 1990 reported the results of 159 esophagogastric anastomoses using the EEA instrument. When performed intrathoracically, minor anastomotic leakage occurred in 9.4% (5/53) of the cases, as opposed to 26.4% (28/106) when constructed antesternally. Anastomotic stenosis occurred in 2 cases (3.8%) intrathoracic and 8 cases (7.5%) antesternal.

In 1989, Fekete reported on 400 esophageal anastomoses performed with the EEA and ILS stapling instruments over a 6-year period. Of the 400 procedures, 268 were esophagogastrostomy, 83 esophagojejunostomy, and 49 esophagocolostomy. The average incidence of leakage and stenosis was 7% and 8%, respectively. No death due to leakage occurred following resection for benign disease. In 1992, Fekete's series' results extended to 1000 esophageal resections with stapled anastomoses performed over a 13-year period.

In 1987, Huang published results of 575 cases of esophagogastric anastomoses performed with a circular anastomosing instrument produced in China, similar to the EEA and ILS stapling instruments in that it places a double staggered circular row of B-shaped staples. The incidence of anastomotic leaks was 1.3% (8/575) compared with 5.6% (20/355) found in manual anastomoses performed in 355 cases before 1980. The occurrence of anastomotic stricture was 1.9%. From mid-1985 to April 1988, they performed 313 intrathoracic stapled anastomoses and reported no leaks.

A review of 221 esophagogastric anastomoses were used by McManus (1990) during a 9-year period to compare hand-sutured and stapled techniques. Of the 122 sutured anastomoses, there were 21 (17.2%) occurrences of leaks. However, there was a significant decrease to 7.1% (7/99) in stapled anastomoses, with a further decrease to 3% (2/69) if the stapled anastomosis required no reinforcing sutures. The incidence of malignant strictures was similar in both groups, but benign strictures were more prevalent in the stapled (13/99 [13%]) group than in the sutured (2/122 [1.6%]) group. The series did not show an increase in stricture rate where gross leakage had been demonstrated. Although the role that leakage plays in stricture formation has not been determined, it was suggested that microleakage through the single row of staples found in the SPTU instrument vs the double row of staples in the EEA instrument may be likely to increase subsequent stricture formation.

MECHANICAL SUTURES IN OPERATIONS ON THE ESOPHAGUS AND GASTROESOPHAGEAL JUNCTION BY ENDOLUMINAL AND INTRACAVITARY ENDOSCOPY

Since the predominant portion of the esophagus is located in the posterior mediastinum, between the right and left chest cavities, this segment can be approached through either the hemithorax or the mediastinum. For reasons of exposure, technical ease, and safety, the transthoracic (open or videoendoscopic) route is preferred over a mediastinal approach, which, by anatomical necessity, advances through a tunnel and is usually characterized by blunt and possibly blind dissection.

The gastroesophageal junction may be approached through the chest or the abdomen and is therefore susceptible to benefit from appropriate thoracoscopic and laparoscopic techniques. The short pharyngoesophageal segment in the neck can be explored through intraluminal endoscopy, just like the thoracoabdominal segments of the esophagus. However, operations that require mobilization of the entire circumference can only be performed through an open cervical approach.

Evolution from the traditional open exposure of the thoracic esophagus and the gastroesophageal junction to a videoendoscopically guided or assisted approach is a logical progression. However, the conversion to a reduced access in operations on the esophagus has to safeguard the usual criteria of sound surgical technique, as well as ensure optimal short- and long-term outcomes, especially in operations for cancer. It also must demonstrate that it is of real benefit to the patient, during his or her hospital stay and immediate postoperative course.

Here we consider only the operations that can be performed with the use of mechanical sutures. However, the field of application of videoendoscopic procedures for the esophagus extends to many endoluminal procedures, as well as to antireflux operations and those used to correct mobility abnormalities. The optical systems and instrumentation are essentially comparable to those used for pulmonary surgery, with the addition of circular anastomosing staplers. The esophagoscope is of great importance as a guide by transillumination from inside. Collapse of the lung on the side of the operative approach is essential with the use of endotracheal double-lumen tubes.

ZENKER'S DIVERTICULOESOPHAGOSTOMY (ENDOLUMINAL MARSUPIALIZATION)

Of the various accepted treatments of a symptomatic Zenker's diverticulum, resection and cricomyotomy or diverticulopexy and cricomyotomy through a left cervicotomy have been standard operations in the surgical repertoire. The minimally invasive, endoscopic, sutureless division of the septum between diverticulum and esophagus through an endoluminal approach has always appeared as an elegant and promising solution. However, the technical means used to achieve transection of the septum and sealing of the diverticular and esophageal walls (e.g., electrocautery and laser coagulation) did not provide the necessary safeguards to make this a widely used technique. As the GIA instrument became available in the late 1960s, Mark Ravitch suggested that a specially constructed GIA instrument would be ideal for the endoluminal approach. However, the small number of patients who would have benefited from such an instrument did not provide the manufacturer with the motivation to undertake the necessary research and development. Changing circumstances do give rise to new incentives and perspectives! With the creation of the ENDO GIA instrument for thoracoscopic and laparoscopic purposes, the dream instrument for the endoscopic treatment of a hypopharyngeal diverticulum became available—(as a by-product). Without any knowledge of Ravitch's earlier suggestion, Collard, Otte, and Kestens from Brussels have used the ENDO GIA stapler most ingeniously for the purpose of transecting the diverticular-esophageal septum and sealing the lips on each side of this transection with triple rows of staples. Since the upper respiratory and digestive passages may become very crowded with the various instruments that are required, the jet ventilation technique for anesthesia—possibly through a small transtracheal catheter—is recommended. In this fashion, the anesthesia function is safely separated from the operative activities and accidental dislocation of an endotracheal tube is avoided. In addition, the risk of oropharyngeal trauma due to a plethora of instruments is reduced to a minimum. Collard and colleagues have used a double-lipped, stationary Weerda laryngoscope that allows adaptation of its two lips to the configuration of the patient's pharynx. The ENDO GIA 30 stapler is then introduced into the pharynx through the passage created by the Weerda laryngoscope, and the instrument forks are placed across the esophagodiverticular spur.

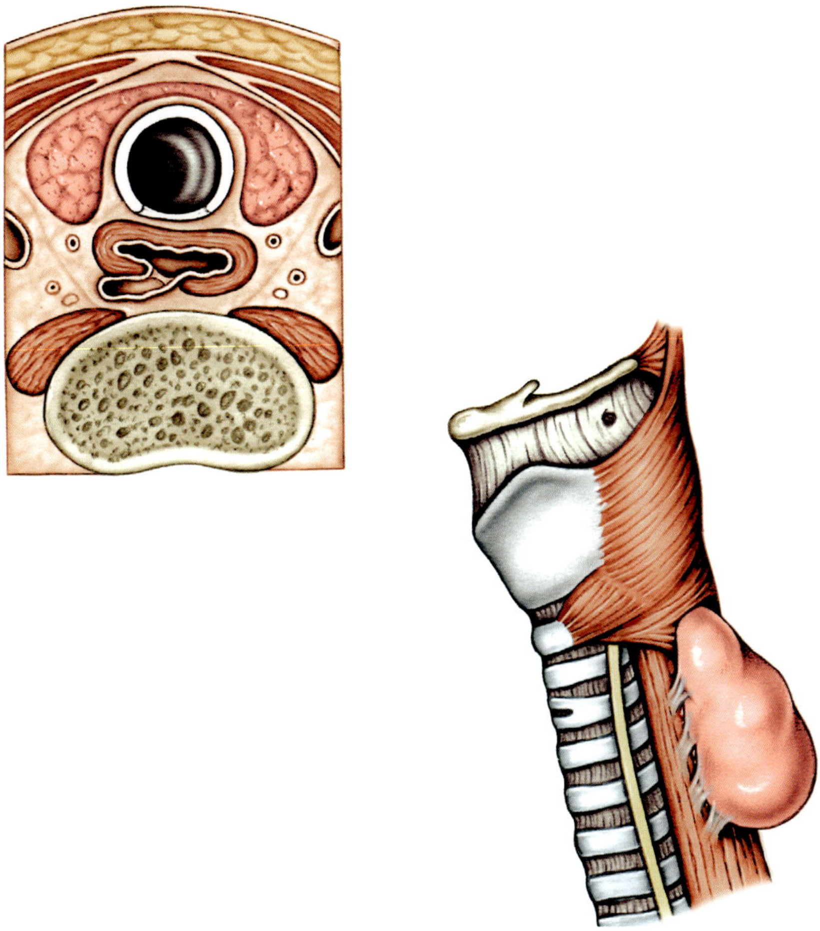

Figure IIIE-1,A,B: The Zenker's, or hypopharyngeal, diverticulum protrudes posteriorly at the level of or through the upper fibers of the cricopharyngeous muscle in the transition zone between the hypopharynx and esophagus. Due to the course of the esophagus in the neck, it is usually directed more into the left prevertebral space, although its ostium is in the posterior wall of the tubular pharyngoesophageal junction. The anatomical details and the attachments between the posterior esophageal and anterior diverticular walls make the endoluminal procedure possible. As a fringe benefit, the transection of the septum also accomplishes a cricomyotomy if the diverticulum extends inferiorly over a sufficient distance. For small diverticula, which require only a single application of the ENDO GIA 30 instrument, Collard has found that enough circular cricopharyngeous muscle remains intact distal to the diverticuloesophagostomy to deny relief of spasm. In these patients, an open approach with diverticulectomy and full cricopharyngomyotomy remains the operation of choice.

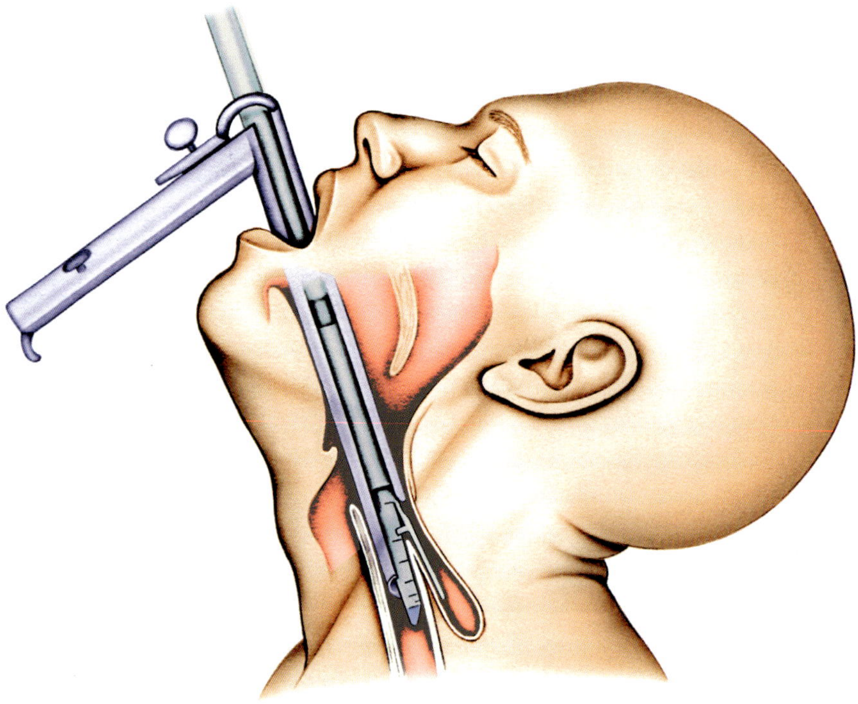

Figure IIIE-1,C: The endoscope and ENDO GIA instrument are introduced transorally.

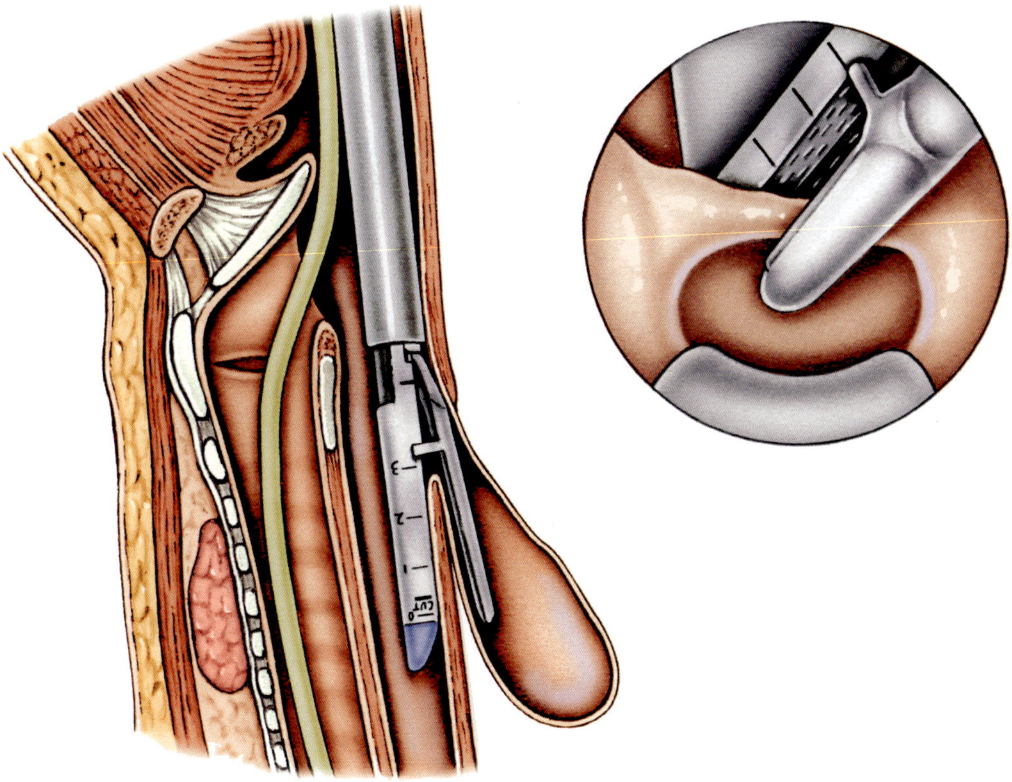

Figure IIIE-1,D,E: The ENDO GIA 30 instrument is positioned with the anvil in the diverticulum and the cartridge in the esophageal lumen. The crotch of the instrument is advanced against the spur, and the instrument is closed and activated.

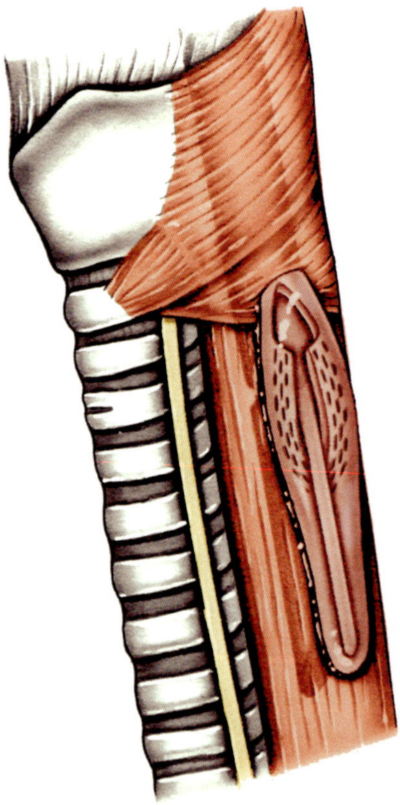

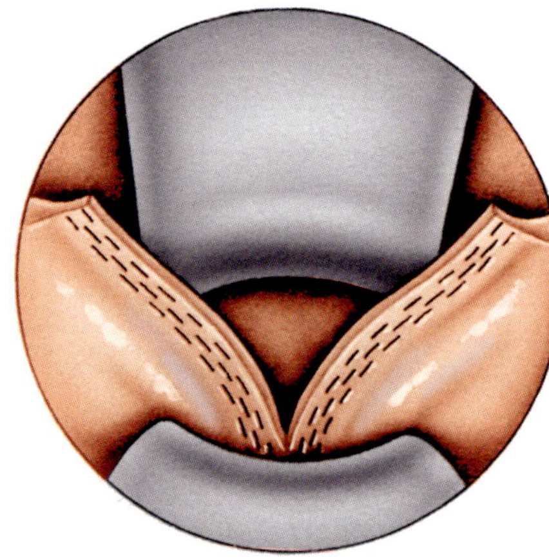

Figure IIIE-1,F,G: Three rows of staples are delivered on each side of the transection, and the sealed edges of the septum are retracted in an open "V" fashion by the pull of the cricopharyngeal muscle.

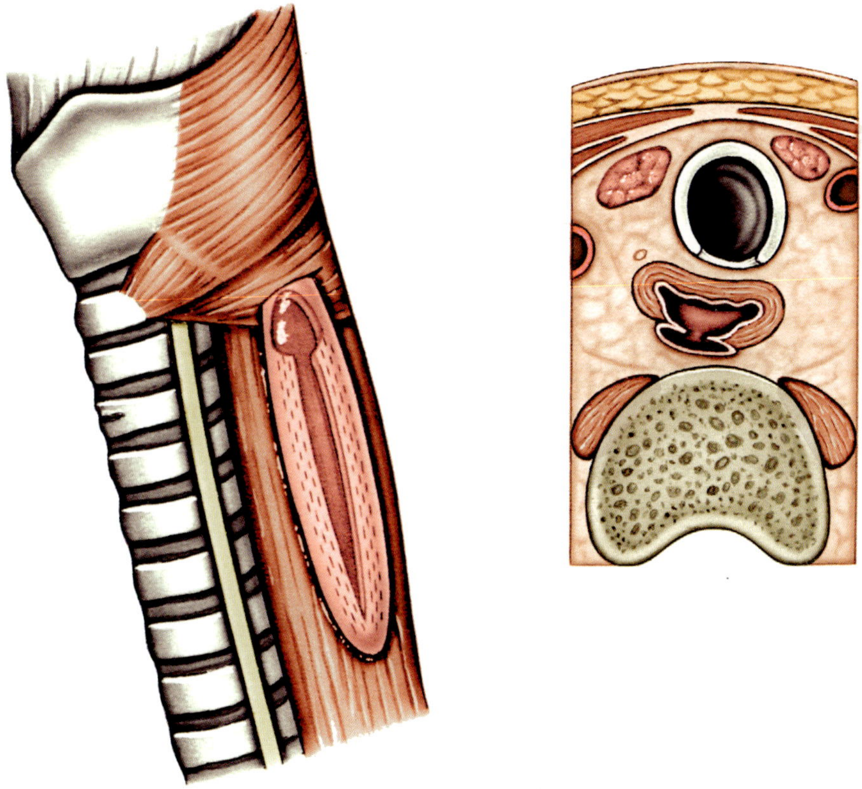

Figure IIIE-1,H,I: The usual, moderate-to-large diverticulum requires the use of a second application of the ENDO GIA 30 stapler across the remaining spur or the ENDO GIA 60 instrument used initially in a single application. As the edges retract further with the pull of the annular musculature, a common cavity and open lumen between the esophagus and diverticulum are created.

THORACOSCOPIC TREATMENT OF ESOPHAGEAL PERFORATION, TUBE PHARYNGOSTOMY, LAPAROSCOPIC GASTROSTOMY, AND FEEDING JEJUNOSTOMY

The replacement of the rigid esophagoscope with a flexible instrument, carrying a much improved light source and providing a clearer, enlarged image, has greatly reduced the incidence of "idiopathic" injuries to the esophagus during diagnostic and foreign-body retrieval endoluminal procedures. However, the incidence of perforations has not been completely eliminated—the esophageal wall remains vulnerable to the combined ill effect of a forceful diagnostic endeavor and a pre-existing condition weakening its integrity. In addition, dietary indiscretions such as in Boerhaave's syndrome, sharp foreign bodies, and penetrating and blunt injuries (Figure III-2) remain a constant liability. However, the association of endoluminal and intracavitary endoscopy has greatly improved the repair and the prognosis of esophageal perforations if they are diagnosed without delay. Furthermore, the temporary exclusion, in continuity, of the restored segment from saliva and acid or bilious reflux with linear, transverse staple lines above and below the repair, favors primary healing without stricture formation (Figure III-11).

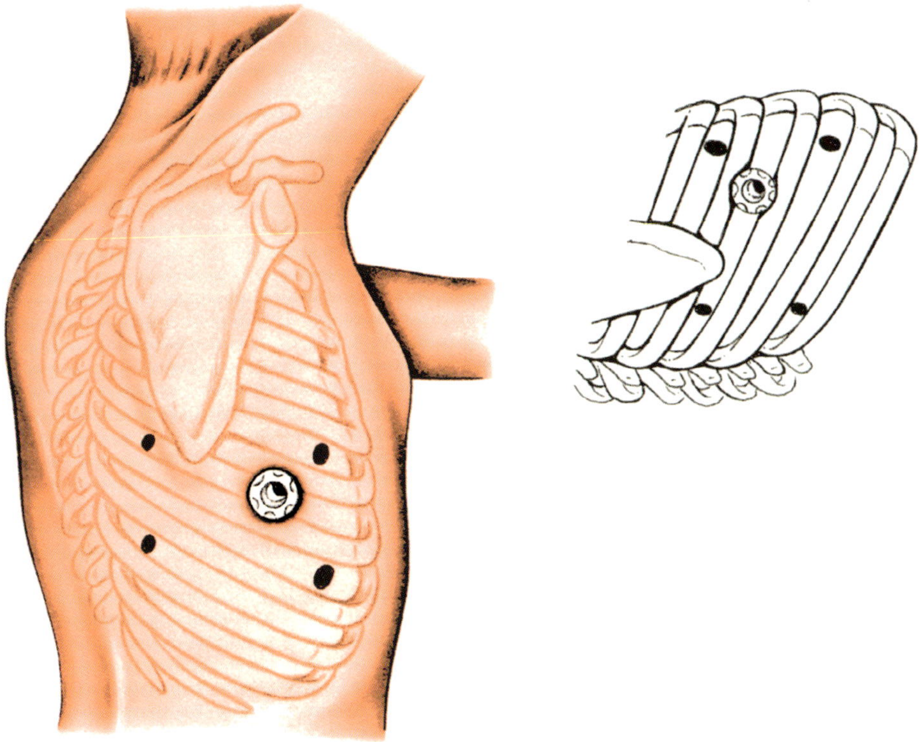

Figure IIIE-2,A: For a right thoracoscopic approach, the endoscope is placed into the fifth ICS-midaxillary line and port sites for the various instruments are established in the fourth and sixth ICS-AAL, as well as in the fifth and seventh ICS-PAL.

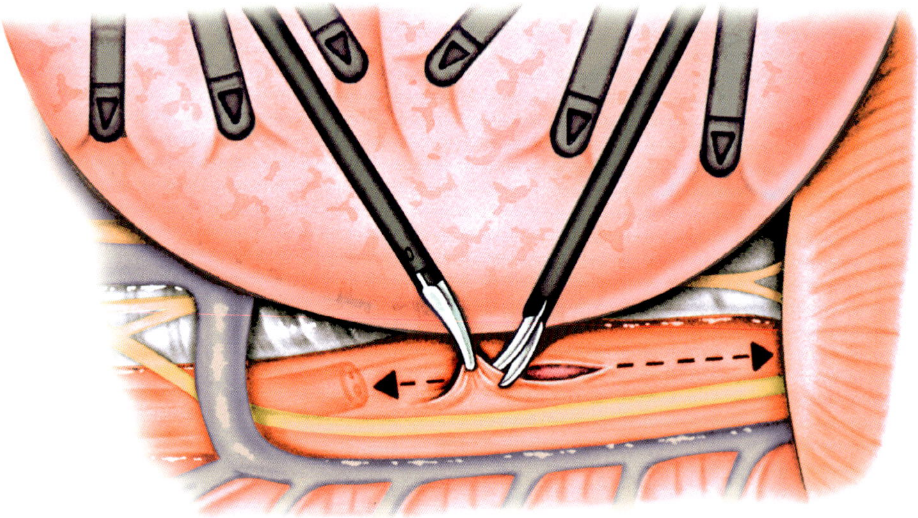

Figure IIIE-2,B: With the endoluminal endoscope in place to help with the identification of the esophagus and of the perforation by transillumination, the mediastinum is opened widely in a superior and inferior direction. The perforation is repaired with interrupted sutures. In this case, the diagnosis was prompt and therefore T-tube drainage, as shown in Figure III-11,A is not indicated.

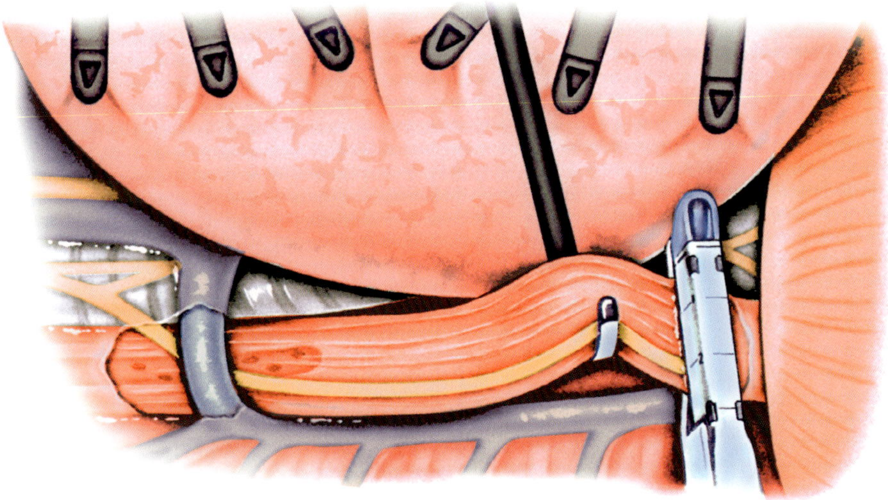

Figure IIIE-2,C: The esophagoscope is replaced by an intraluminally "dangling" suction tube, proximal to the repair, placed through a lateral pharyngostomy. The esophagus distal to the repair is elevated circumferentially. The ENDO TA instrument is placed transversely, across the esophageal wall, just above the GE junction, then closed and activated. In a small, clean perforation we do not place a temporary staple line proximal to the repair, but we do rely on the pharyngostomy tube to aspirate the saliva. The handling of the vagus nerves is a matter of surgical judgment; if the patient's condition is stable, the nerves would be elevated from the esophagus and the ENDO TA stapler would be positioned below the nerves.

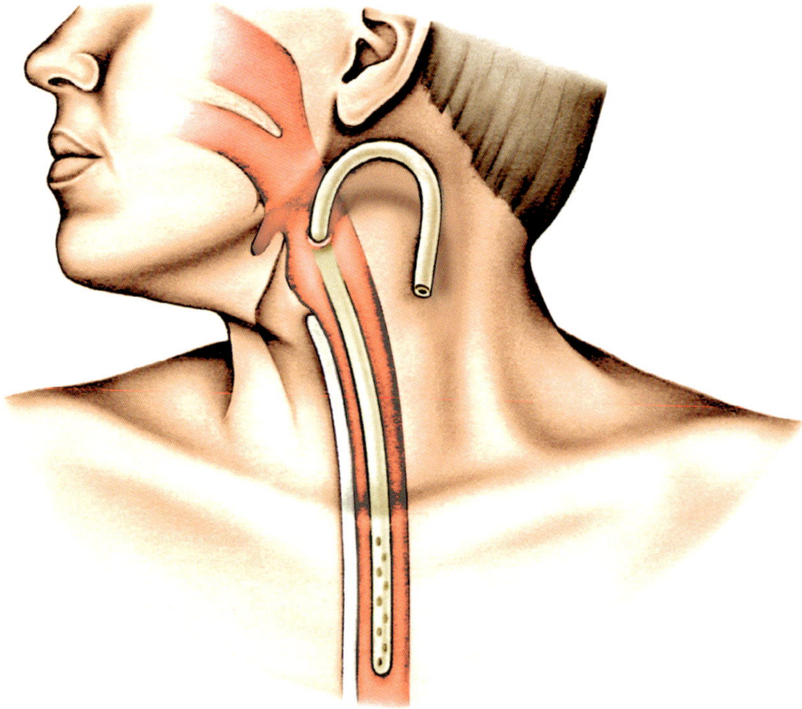

Figure IIIE-2,D: Rather than performing a debilitating, fully diverting, cervical esophagostomy that will require formal repair later, a lateral suction tube pharyngostomy, placed percutaneously and through the lower pole of the pyriform sinus into the esophagus behind the larynx, will prevent the saliva from seeping down. At this level, the pyriform sinus is practically subcutaneous and the optimal trajectory for the ostomy tube, anterior to all the vessel compartments, can be selected through bimanual palpation, with one index finger in the patient's throat, behind and lateral to the larynx, and the index finger of the other hand on the skin, just below the mandible. The two fingers should palpate what is essentially skin and pharyngeal mucosa between them. The suction tube is then placed through a stab wound, carefully initiated onto the endopharyngeal finger, and the tube is advanced into the pharynx and down into the esophagus, behind the larynx.

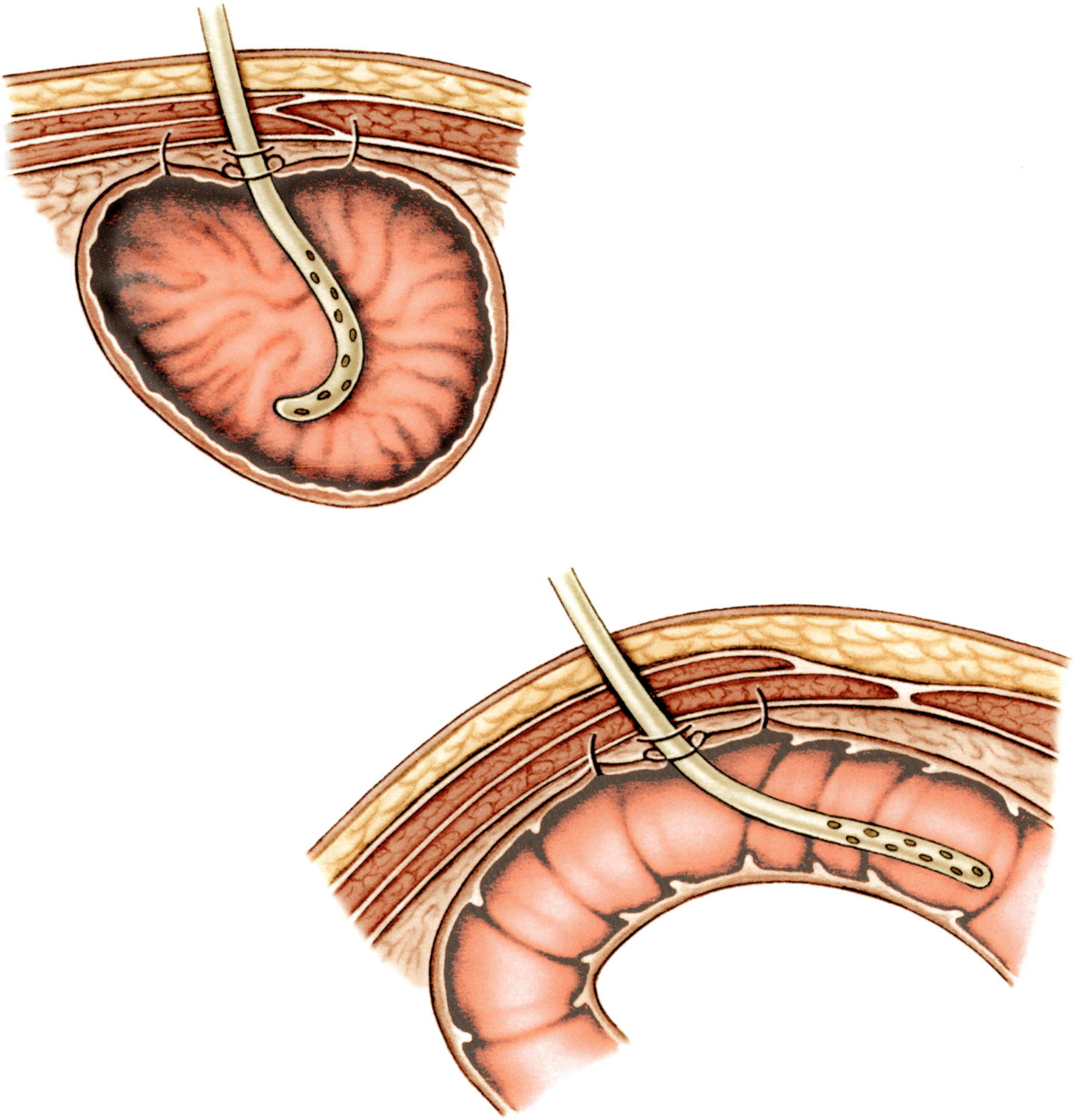

Figure IIIE-2,E,F: A gastrostomy is then established by laparoscopic techniques. Similarly, a feeding jejunostomy is placed at the same time, by laparoscopic means. Patients who have suffered an esophageal perforation are often malnourished because of underlying disease. A jejunostomy provides a more safe way to ensure nutrition than the more cumbersome and hazardous venous hyperalimentation.

EPIPHRENIC DIVERTICULECTOMY

Traditionally, epiphrenic diverticula are treated by resection through a left thoracotomy, extramucosal myotomy of the lower esophageal segment, and anterior fundoplication if gastroesophageal reflux is part of the clinical picture.

Symptomatic parabronchial traction diverticula are treated by closure of the neck with sutures or staples and excision. This can now be accomplished by videoendoscopic techniques using the ENDO GIA stapler. Peracchia from Milan has suggested and used the same operative technique for the treatment of epiphrenic diverticula. In order to assess lower esophageal sphincter or segment activity, all candidates for a thoracoscopic epiphrenic diverticulectomy undergo preoperative barium swallow, esophagoscopy, 24-hour esophageal pH monitoring, and manometry. If the lower esophageal segment is hypertensive or fails to relax physiologically, Peracchia and colleagues perform a pneumatic dilation of the GE junction using low-compliance balloons inflated to 10 psi for 1 minute, in preparation for right thoracoscopic diverticulectomy later.

The success of this approach is monitored by gastrografin swallow 7 days later, manometry, and pH studies. If all parameters are favorable, right videoendoscopic thoracic diverticulectomy is performed and the result is examined with esophagograms, esophagoscopy, and esophageal-function studies.

Collard and colleagues recommend this procedure, especially for large diverticula in the elderly or generally debilitated patients. Judging from their results, it appears that this method could become a technique of first choice for most patients. Peracchia and colleagues confirmed this expanded indication through very satisfactory anatomical and functional results obtained 6 to 10 months postoperatively, at the time of their report. One patient had a leak at the staple line that required uneventful repair through a thoracotomy. Dysphagia and frequent episodes of aspiration pneumonia were eliminated. Postoperative gastrografin swallow showed a large locally cavitary lumen, with easy passage of the food bolus into the stomach and no retention of food above the GE junction. Manometry demonstrated a satisfactory reduction of pressure in the proximal esophageal segment.

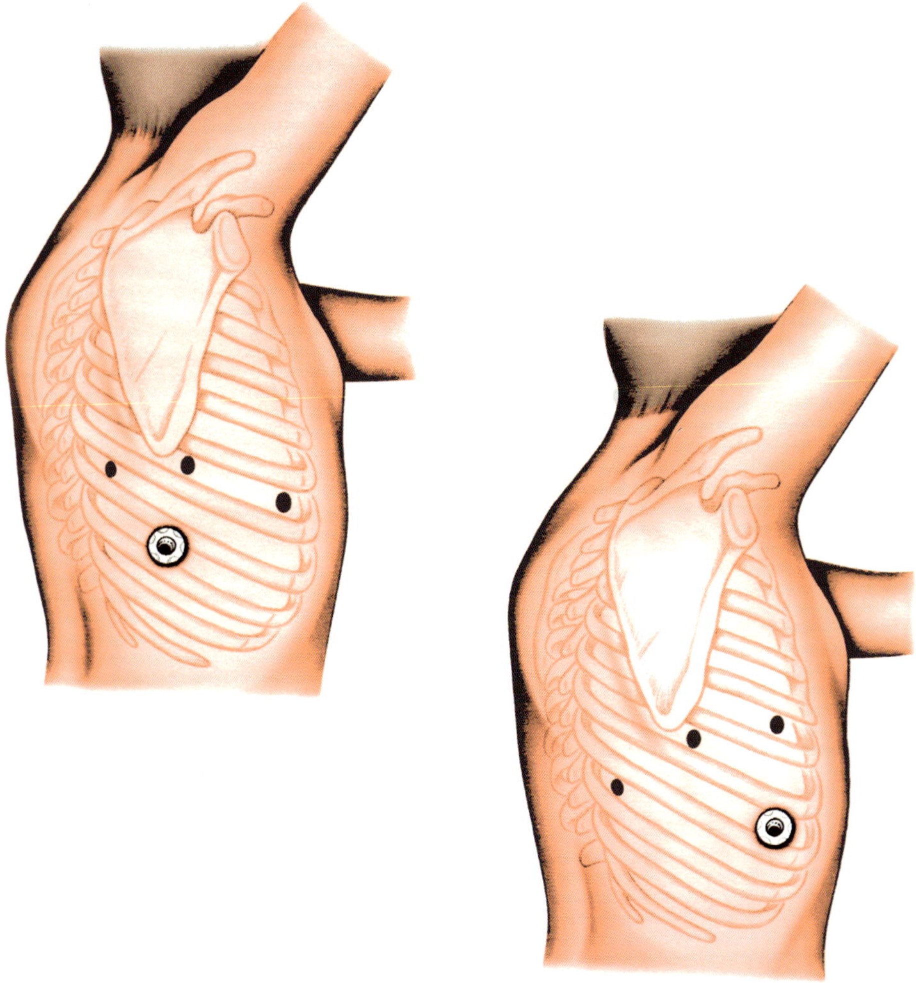

Figure IIIE-3,A,B: The placement of the working ports and the port for the thoracoscope is adapted to the level of the diverticulum.

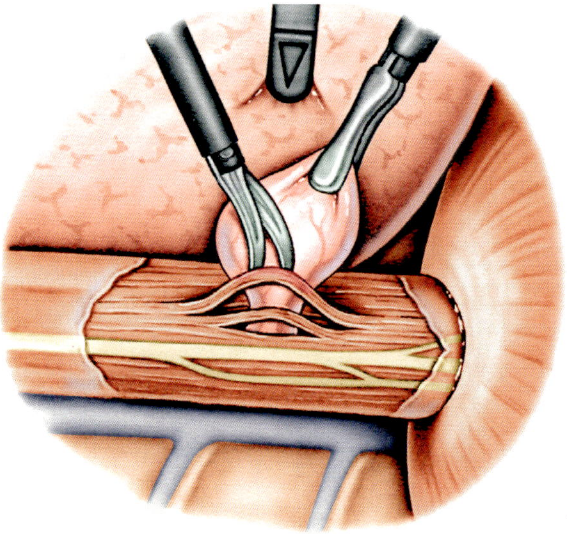

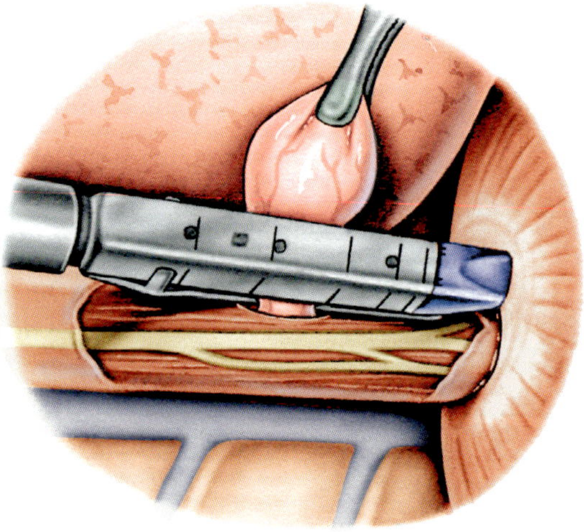

Figure IIIE-3,C: The excision of a low-lying diverticulum is shown. The neck of the diverticulum, regardless of a left- or right-sided outpouching, is usually on the posterior wall of the esophagus, which has to be rotated toward the surgical approach. The diverticulum is grasped, and muscle fibers attached to its base and neck are lifted off with scissor tips.

Figure IIIE-3,D: Following complete liberation of the diverticulum, its neck is closed and transected with the ENDO GIA 30 stapler.

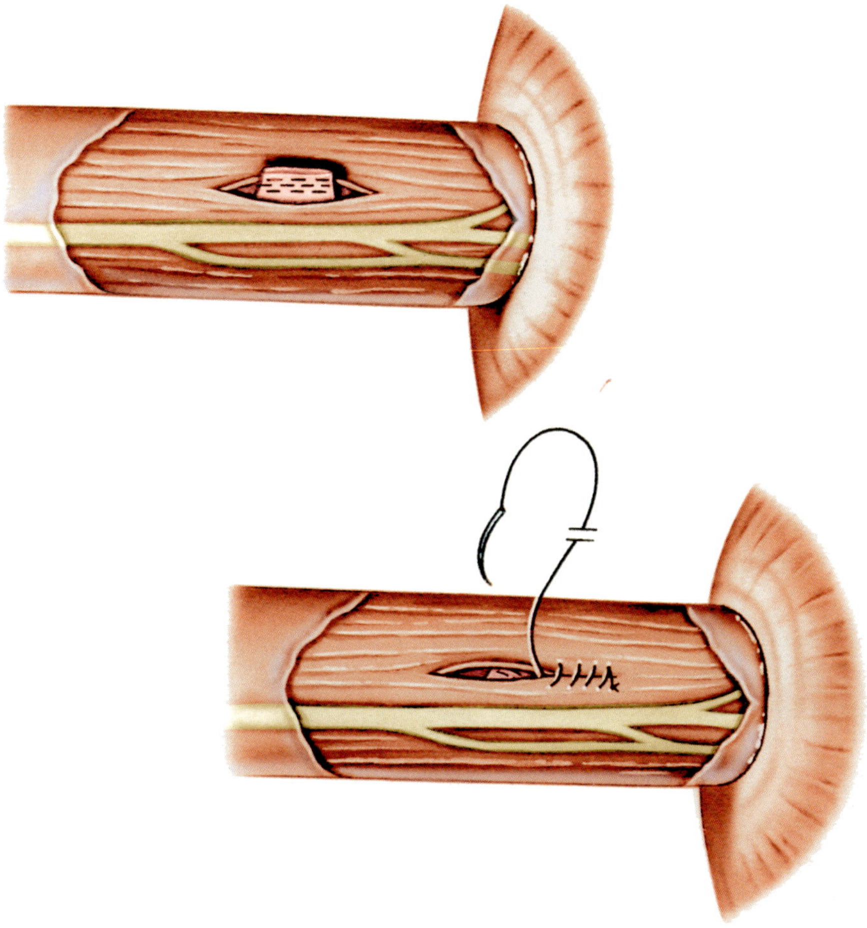

Figure IIIE-3,E,F: The muscle fibers overlying this closure are approximated with a running suture.

ESOPHAGEAL LEIOMYOMECTOMY

In patients with symptomatic leiomyoma of the esophagus, open transthoracic extramucosal enucleation of this benign tumor can now be replaced with a videoendoscopic approach. Intraluminal, intraoperative esophagoscopy is again essential since it helps with delineation of the level and extent of the tumor, mobilization of the surrounding esophagus, and control of mucosal integrity at the end of the operation. Collapse of the ipsilateral lung with a double-lumen endotracheal tube is again mandatory.

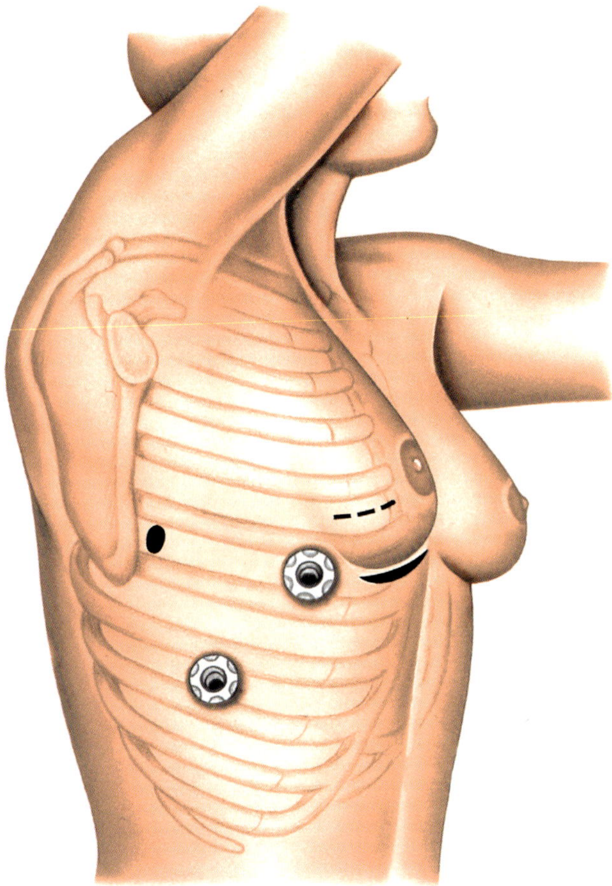

Figure IIIE-4,A: The placement of the thoracic ports and utility incision used by Roviaro and colleagues from Milan is shown. Two working ports in the fifth intercostal space and the anterior and posterior axillary lines, respectively, as well as a seventh intercostal and midaxillary port for the thoracoscope, are used. In women, the skin incision for the anterior fourth intercostal utility incision is placed somewhat lower in the submammary fold.

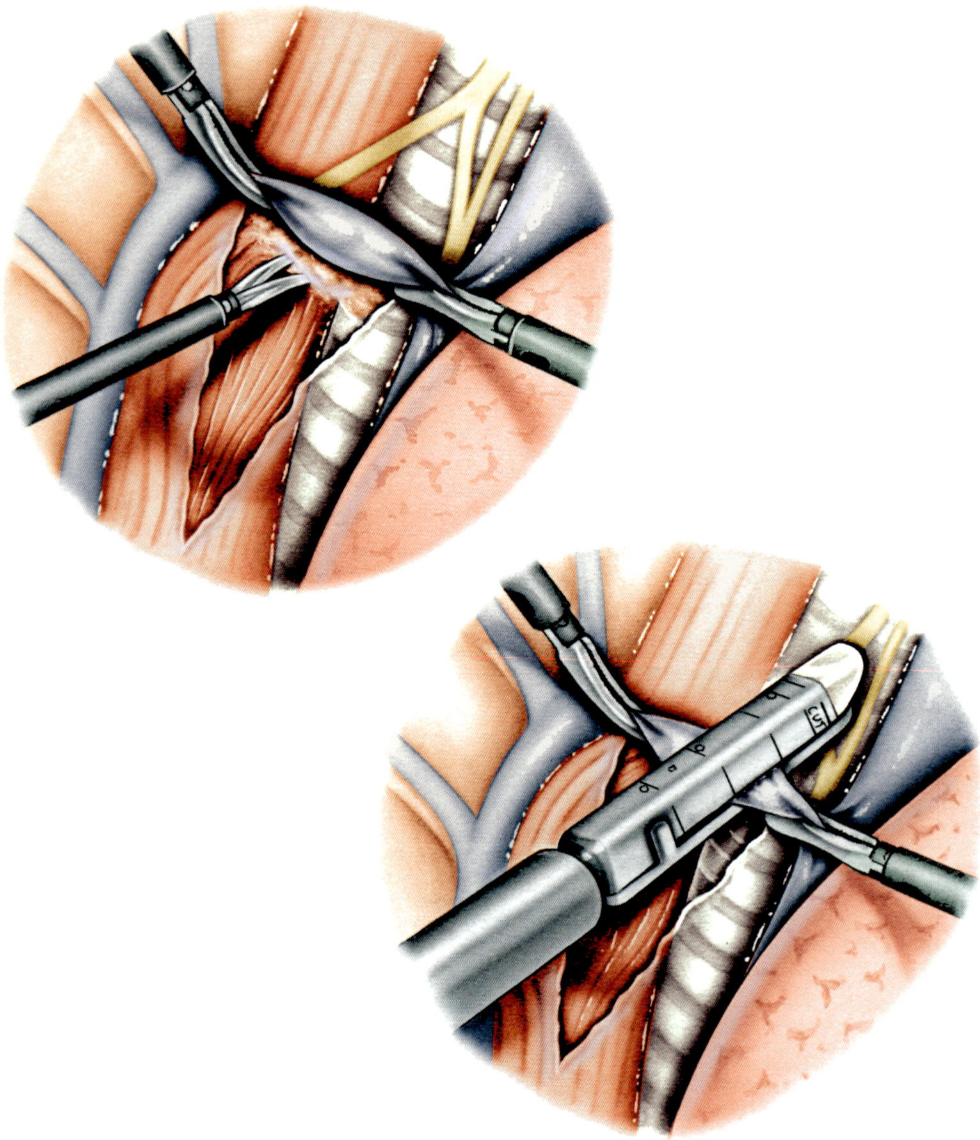

Figure IIIE-4,B,C: A right-sided approach is shown. (The operation for a left-sided leiomyoma, depending on its location, is somewhat limited by the arch of the aorta and may require primary open thoracotomy). With the right lung collapsed and held with a retractor through the utility incision, the mediastinal pleura is opened over the esophageal segment containing the tumor. If the leiomyoma is located in the proximal esophagus, the right hemiazygos vein has to be cleared off the esophagus. Following complete circumferential liberation, the vein is stapled on both sides of its transection with the vascular ENDO GIA stapler.

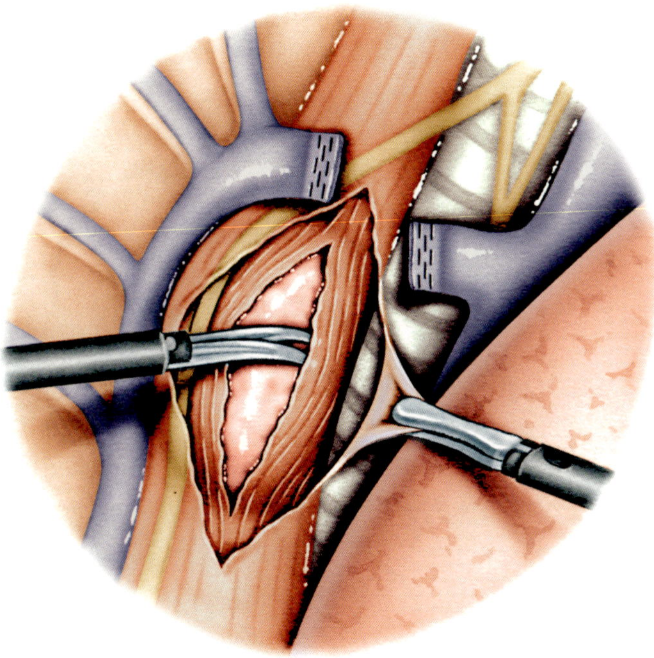

Figure IIIE-4,D: With transillumination by intraluminal esophagoscopy, the tumor size is defined and the esophageal muscular wall is incised longitudinally over the full length of the leiomyoma.

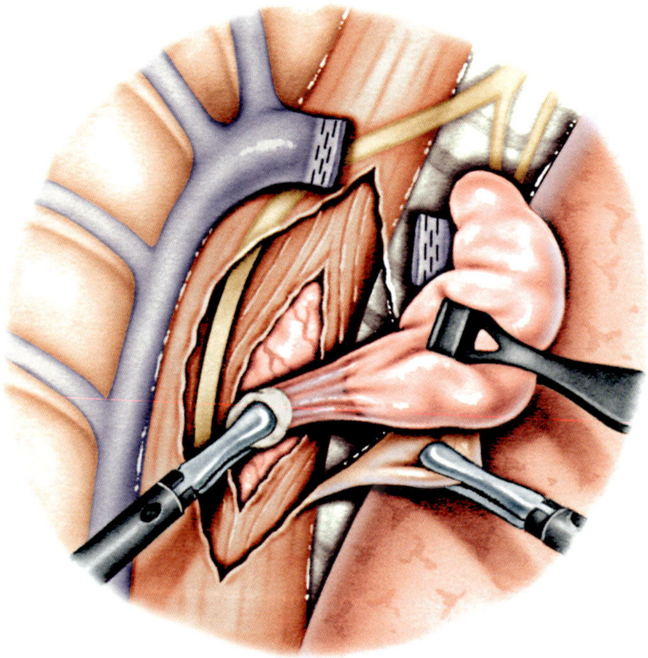

Figure IIIE-4,E: Enucleation and extramucosal dissection of the tumor are carried out with closed scissor tips and a Kuttner dissector and gentle spreading of the scissor tips and occasional cutting of a strand or adhesion. The specimen is held with a Babcock clamp and removed after complete liberation through the utility incision.

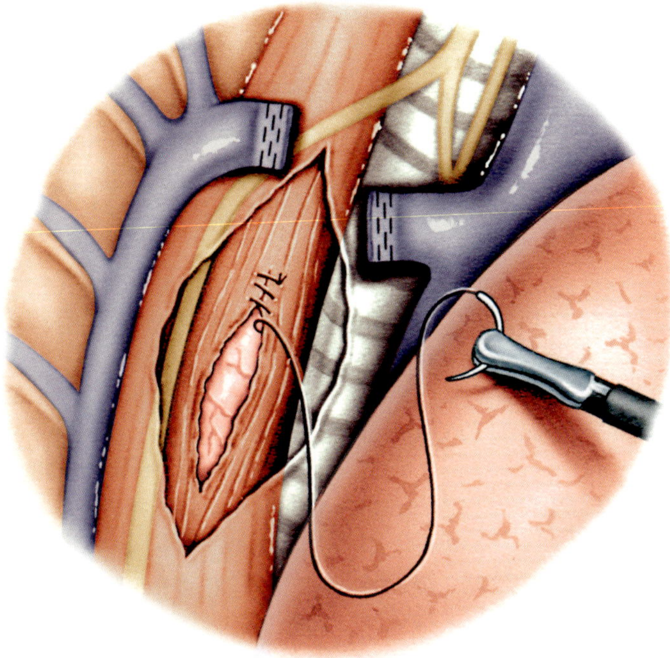

Figure IIIE-4,F: Following complete removal of the tumor and intraluminal endoscopic verification of mucosal integrity, the muscular incision is closed with a running suture. Peracchia and Roviaro consider this step as essential, since pseudodiverticular bulging of the mucosa had been observed in a patient in whom the muscle layer had not been approximated. If the mucosa is injured and this injury is small and clearly visible and reachable, repair can be attempted by thoracoscopically guided means. In most cases, the better part of valor would probably dictate open repair through a minithoracotomy, the level of which can be determined by transthoracic illumination, directly overlying the operative site.

THORACIC ESOPHAGECTOMY

When a total thoracic esophagectomy is planned, with construction of a substitute organ from the abdomen and anastomosis to the pharyngoesophageal segment in the neck, the transthoracic esophagectomy can be safely accomplished using a videoendoscopic approach. This circumvents the intraoperative and postoperative interference with cardiopulmonary function of open thoracotomy and obviates compression and partial intermittent dislocation of the heart, as well as the more traumatic dissection and tunnel vision, if the mostly blunt transhiatal esophagectomy is performed. The visual magnification afforded by the various optical systems, including the more recently available three-dimensional viewing, provides a better image of the primary lesion and the local and regional node involvement, especially if this exploratory phase is bolstered by intraluminal inspection with a flexible fiberoptic esophagoscope. In addition, the pliable tip of the esophagoscope can be used to elevate the esophagus from its longitudinal bed and help with the deep circumferential dissection of this tubular organ. Technically, it is easier to dissect benign and small malignant lesions, especially of the lower half of the esophagus. Collard and colleagues have noted that “en bloc” dissection of larger tumors and nodes around and behind the trachea is difficult to accomplish and that an open approach is preferable, if a soft tissue plane can be developed that is not involved with tumor, during the initial thoracoscopic phase. However, as is so often the case, resection in this area may only be palliative because of adherence to or invasion of the carina, left main stem bronchus, or aorta by tumor. In these cases, the less invasive maneuver of initial thoracoscopy, followed by palliative resection, which is guided by endoscopic inspection and staging, surgical judgment, and restraint are preferable to the more traumatic open thoracotomy. Videoendoscopically guided brachytherapy for residual tumor, external beam radiotherapy, and retrosternal bypass with stomach or large bowel are acceptable alternative treatments in such cases. In these patients, laparoscopic staging of possible abdominal metastases not detected by CT scan should precede laparotomy for creation of a substitute organ, using essentially the same instruments as for thoracoscopy. If metastases below the diaphragm are found, palliation should consist of radiotherapy only, with or without placement of an endoluminal prosthesis.

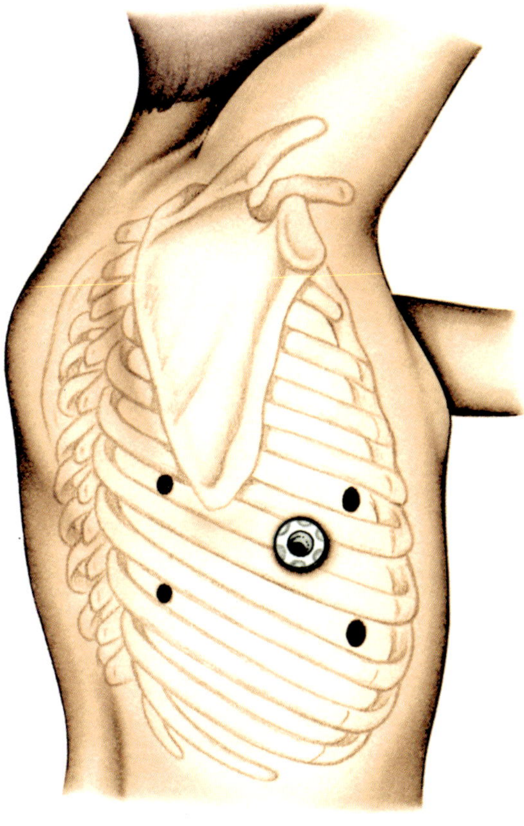

Figure IIIE-5,A: The patient is in the left lateral decubitus position, with the right side up. The right arm is elevated and rotated anteriorly to keep the axilla free for an additional port. The placement of the thoracic ports used by Peracchia, Rosati, and colleagues is shown. Basically, the scheme represents a horizontal "X," extending from the anterior axillary to the midscapular line, at the fourth and sixth intercostal spaces anteriorly and the fifth and seventh spaces posteriorly. The thoracoscope port is placed at the intersection of both lines, which is the fifth intercostal space and midaxillary line.

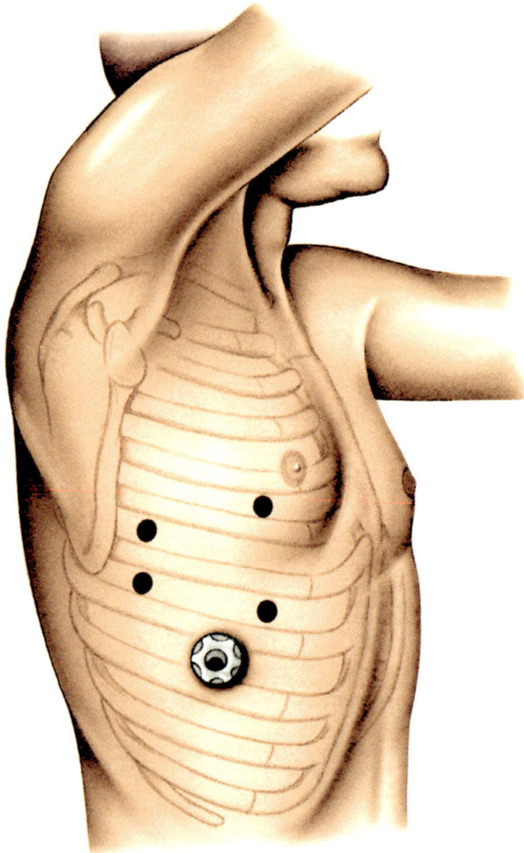

Figure IIIE-5,B: The placement scheme used by Gossot and Celerier from Paris also provides for two anterior ports for lung retraction and two working ports in the posterior axillary or lateral scapular line and the fifth and sixth intercostal spaces. The scope and camera are placed into the midaxillary line and the seventh intercostal space.

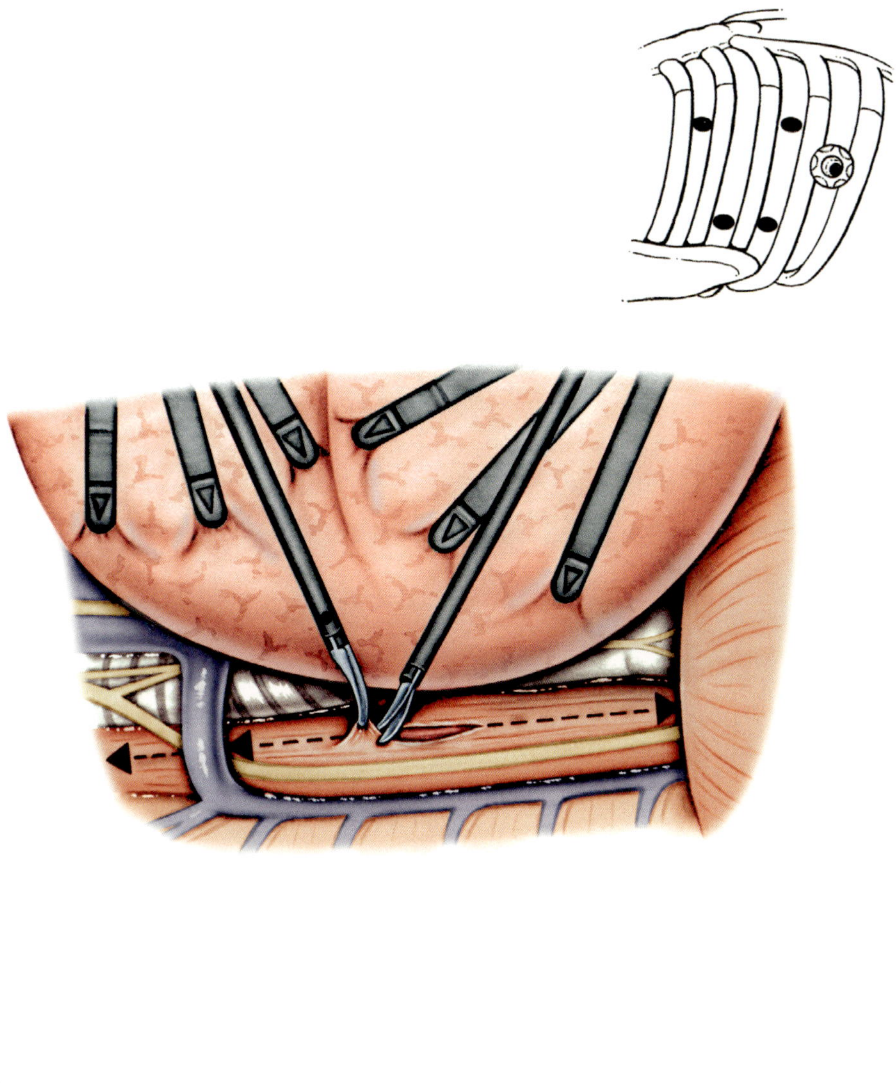

Figure IIIE-5,C: Correct placement of the double-lumen endotracheal tube is of utmost importance to facilitate gentle progressive compression of the collapsed right lung. This collapse is enhanced by aspiration of air from the right main bronchus and, if needed, moderate CO_2 insufflation into the right hemithorax. The esophagus is identified from within its lumen, ideally with a flexible esophagoscope and transillumination or with a medium size mercury bougie. The mediastinal pleura is grasped, elevated, and incised. This incision is carried superiorly and inferiorly, and the right lateral aspect of the esophagus is laid bare with blunt and sharp dissection using the scissor tips.

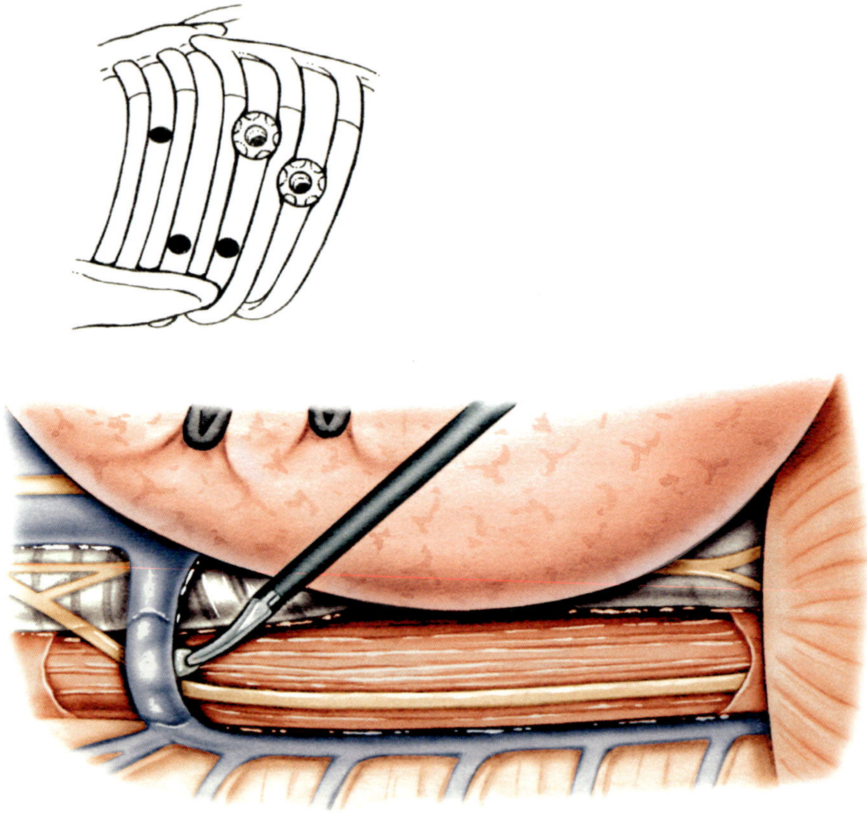

Figure IIIE-5,D: By switching the thoracoscope into the lower anterior port, a dissector placed through the viewing port is used to elevate the posterior aspect of the azygos vein.

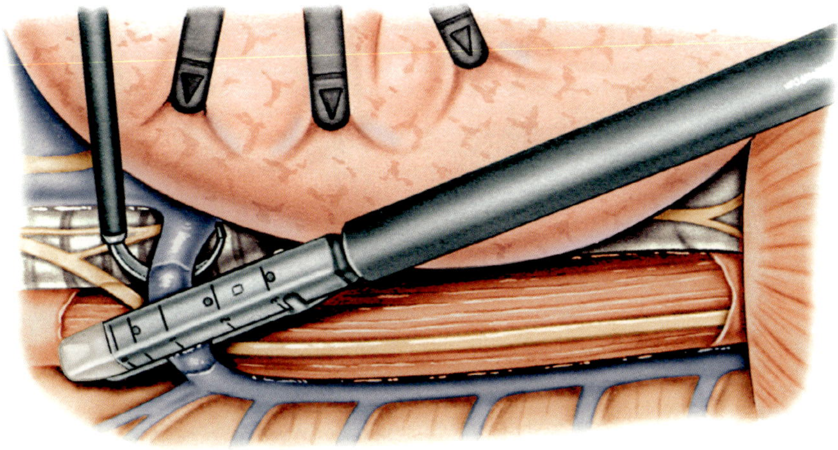

Figure IIIE-5,E: The circumferentially liberated right hemiazygos vein is elevated with a curved mini-retractor and engaged into the open vascular ENDO GIA 30. The instrument is closed and activated and both sides of the vein transection are ligated with three staggered rows of staples.

Roviaro and colleagues have noted that manipulations in the apex of the chest—required, for instance, in the excision of a leiomyoma or the mobilization of a bulky esophageal tumor—have resulted in repeated minor injuries to the stubby vein ends, dislocation of some staples. and bothersome bleeding. They prefer, therefore, one anterior and one posterior application of the vascular ENDO TA stapler on the curved hemiazygos vein, leaving the midportion of the vein free for transection by endoscopic scissors. This maneuver leaves a buffer zone between the vein stumps and their respective closures that are removed from direct contact with dissecting instruments.

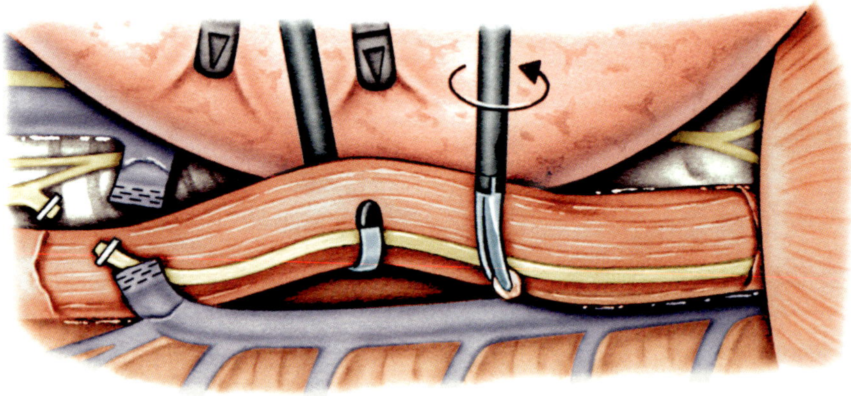

Figure IIIE-5,F: The esophagus is dissected circumferentially in its mid-downward course with a blunt dissector and the closed tips of the scissors. In this dissection, some advantage can be gained by identifying the boundaries of the muscular tube by transillumination and elevating various points of separation from the mediastinal bed with the flexible tip of the endoluminal esophagoscope. In its absence, a soft mercury bougie can be helpful at this stage.

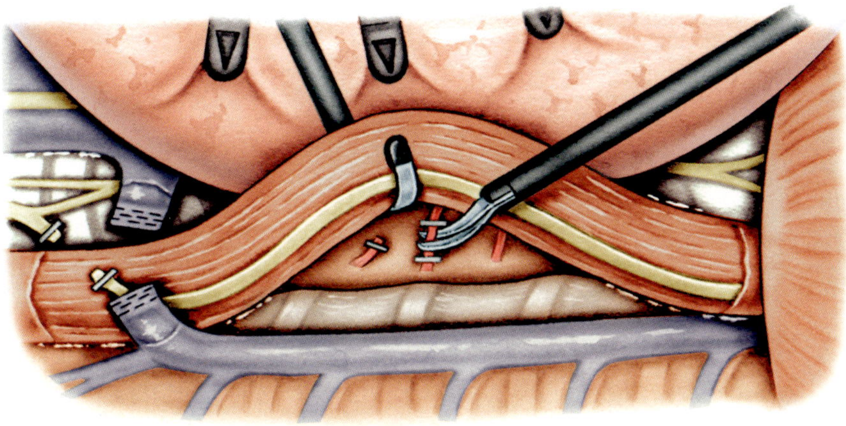

Figure IIIE-5,G: With the esophagoscope or bougie pulled back proximally to provide greater flexibility and the esophagus held elevated with a curved mini-retractor, dissection is extended superiorly and inferiorly all around the organ. Hemostasis is accomplished with clips and electrocautery. The vagus nerves are transected caudad to the respective recurrent laryngeal nerve branches and are included with the future specimen, as are all sympathetic and parasympathetic nerve fibers that may enter or leave a given tumor, as well as all visible lymphatic drainage sites and nodes.

The dissection into the thoracic outlet superiorly and into the diaphragmatic hiatus inferiorly can be incomplete at this point and may be completed through a laparotomy and a neck incision, made for the creation and proximal anastomosis of a substitute organ. The esophagus is temporarily left in place and will be pulled out through the neck incision and used to elevate the attached substitute organ into the neck through the hiatus and the original esophageal bed, unless a retrosternal route is preferred. As this maneuver takes place, the mediastinal passage may be observed with a thoracoscope at the price of returning the patient from a dorsal position to a left lateral decubitus position.

The anastomosis in the neck can be manual or mechanical, using any of the appropriate techniques previously shown.

We do not recommend a laparoscopically guided or assisted substitute organ creation. Although others have done this, the combined thoracoscopy and laparoscopy times add up to a marathon of truly Olympian proportions even in the hands of established champions. The trauma to the patient's homeostasis may well outweigh the benefit of preserving abdominal wall integrity. However, an initial minimal thoracic and abdominal approach, considered as a preliminary step, is based on solid reasoning because it may limit the planned excision and reconstruction to tumor and nodal staging only. A small incision is preferable if it turns out that the tumor and/or nodal metastases are inoperable. Conversely, this argument does not prevail if the operative findings favor the expanded effort of excising tumor and metastatic lymph nodes and commits to the choice and intricate technical details of autologous organ reconstruction. In that situation, our preference goes to extending the preliminary diagnostic and staging thoracoscopy into a full blown excisional procedure, if possible, but to limit the preliminary staging laparoscopy to diagnosis only, and undertaking the creation of the chosen substitute organ through a laparotomy.

BELSEY MARK IV PROCEDURE

The Belsey Mark IV procedure by thoracoscopic technique is indicated in patients who have had previous extensive intra-abdominal operation(s) that would make a laparoscopic Nissen procedure impossible and would turn a laparotomy into a tedious undertaking because of expected adhesions. It should also be considered in patients with a failed Nissen procedure, especially if the gastric wrap has herniated partially or entirely through the hiatus with moderate shortening of the esophagus. The dissection of the deteriorated fundoplication and temporary restoration of normal anatomy is easier and safer from the mediastinum downward.

The Belsey procedure provides reliable anchoring of the fundoplication below the hiatus, especially in patients with moderate esophageal shortening. A Collis-Nissen procedure should be performed (Figure III-20, A to D) if the shortening does not allow the comfortable repositioning of the GE junction below the hiatus following liberation of the esophagus up to and beyond the inferior pulmonary ligament. This operation can be accomplished through a thoracotomy or by thoracoscopy. All patients should have had an esophagoscopy and four quadrant biopsies of the lower esophageal segment to rule out malignant transformation of longstanding esophagitis.

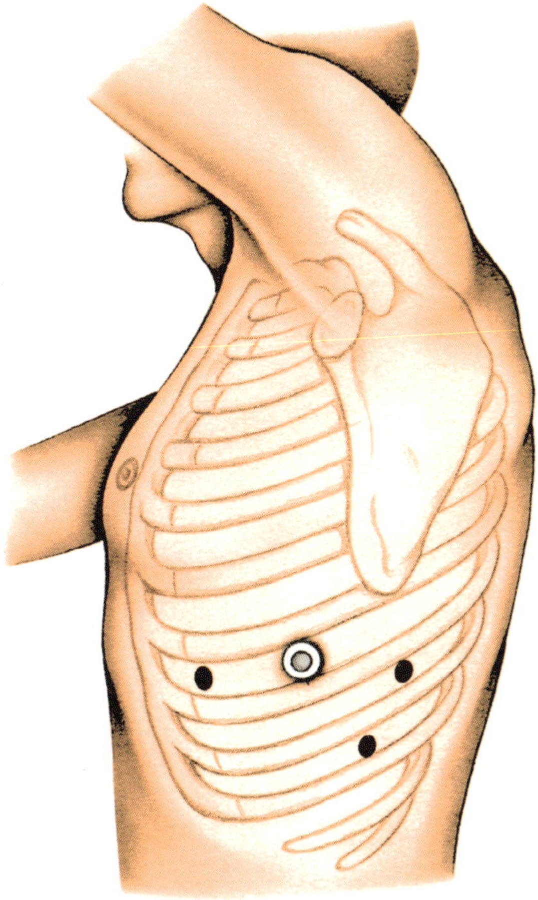

Figure IIIE-6,A: With the left arm elevated to facilitate placement and movement of the thoracoscope and instruments, the endoscope port is placed into the seventh ICS-midaxillary line and instrument ports are established in the seventh ICS-AAL and in the eighth and ninth ICS-PAL or anterior scapular line.

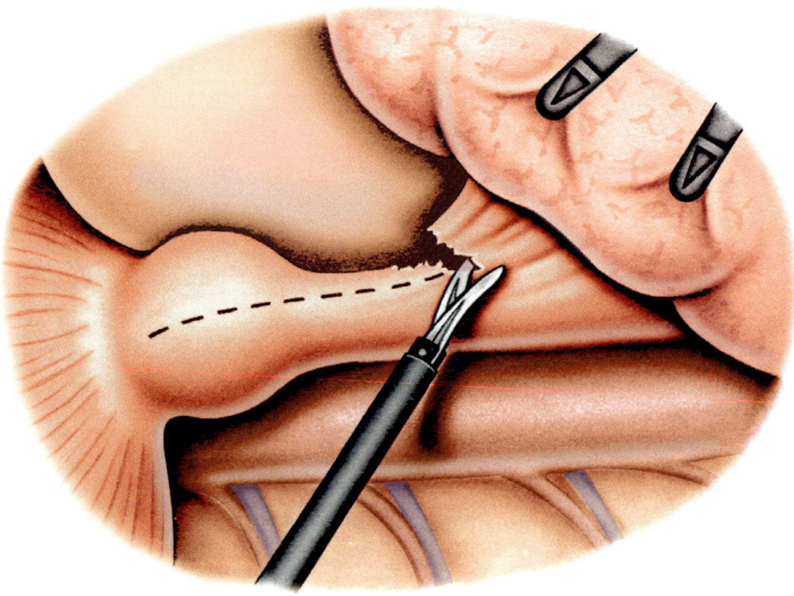

Figure IIIE-6,B: The distal esophagus and cardia are mobilized up to and including the inferior pulmonary ligament. The hernia sac and lower mediastinum are entered through a vertical incision, as indicated by the dotted line.

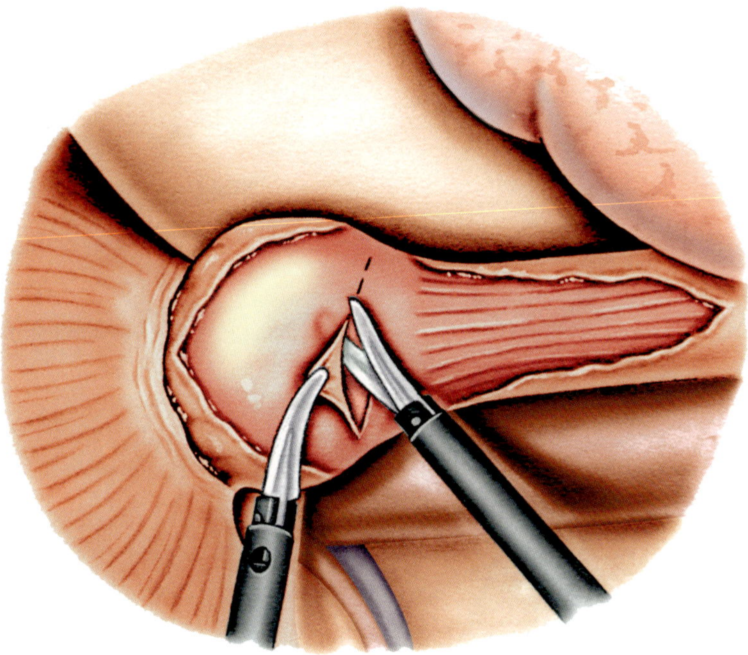

Figure IIIE-6,C: The entire circumference of the cardia is separated from its attachments. This requires division of branches from the inferior phrenic artery laterally and from the left gastric artery posteriorly.

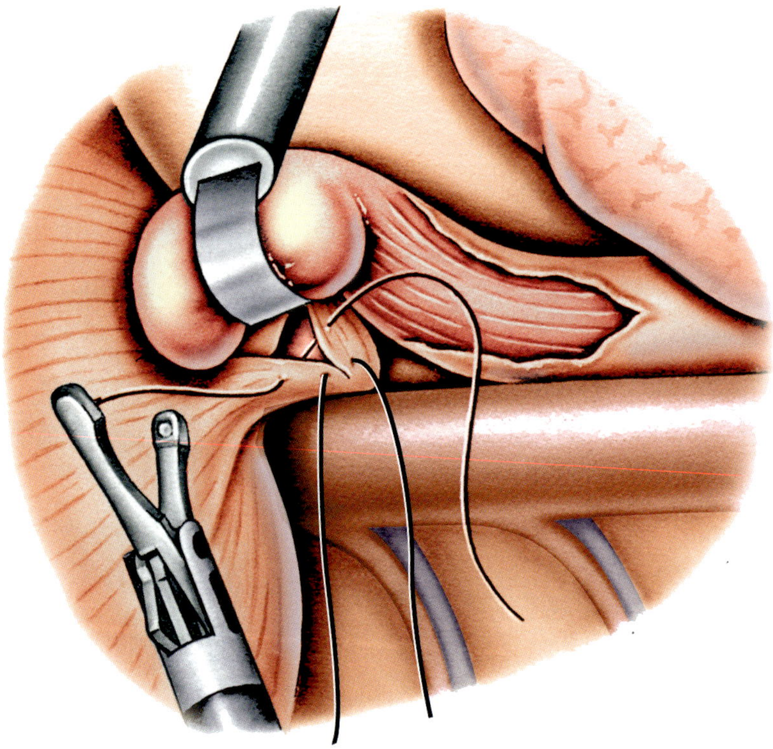

Figure IIIE-6,D: With the GE junction elevated anteriorly, the left and right crural pillars are identified and sutures are placed across the hiatus posteriorly. These sutures are left untied for the time being. However, the caliber of the hiatus is adjusted now by pulling these sutures tight, with a large intraluminal bougie in place, to make sure that the hiatal repair is adequate. Sutures are added, or removed as the case may be, if the repair is too loose or too tight.

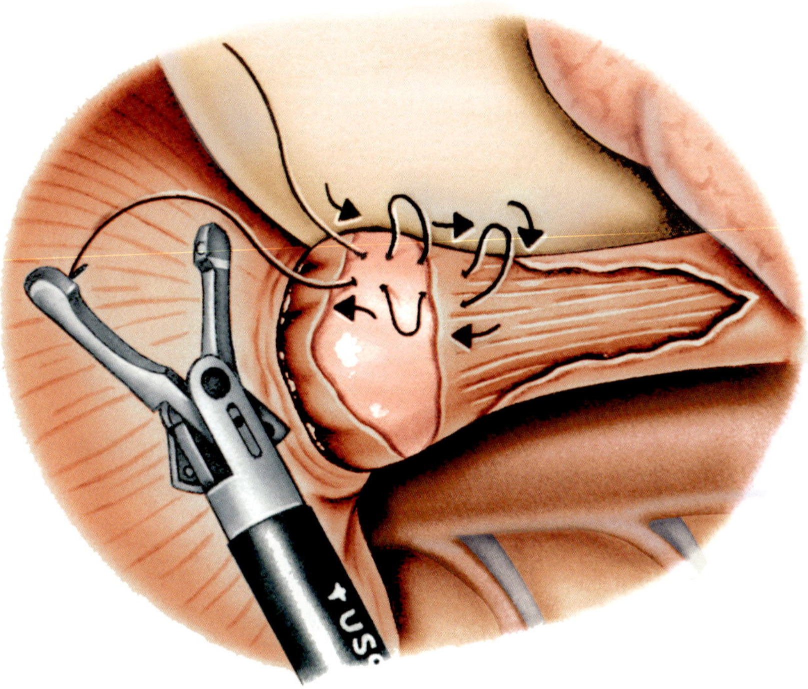

Figure IIIE-6,E: The mobilization of the GE junction is completed down to the pad of fibrofatty tissue that is a constant companion of the cardia. This pad is excised anteriorly and laterally; the vagus nerves that tend to be elevated by this dissection are carefully preserved. The repair of antireflux function is started by placing the first of three mattress sutures between the fundus of the stomach and the esophagus, 2 cm above the GE junction.

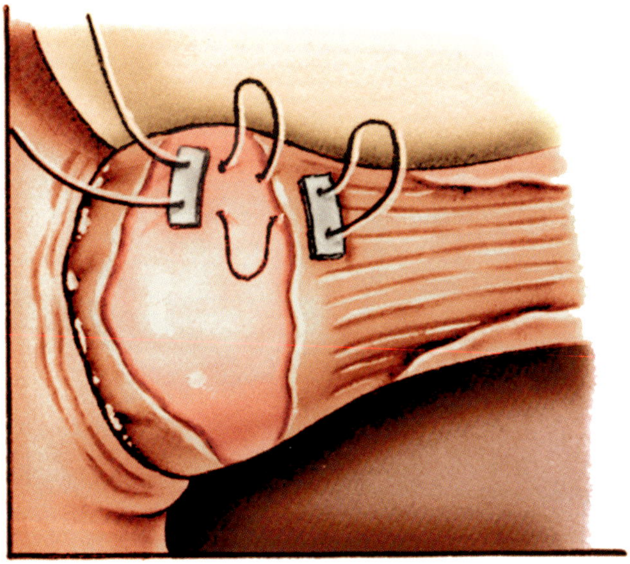

Figure IIIE-6,F: In order to prevent the mattress sutures from cutting through the tissues, especially on the esophageal side, pledgets may be used not only to provide a firm base for the sutures and ties, but also to protect the tissues.

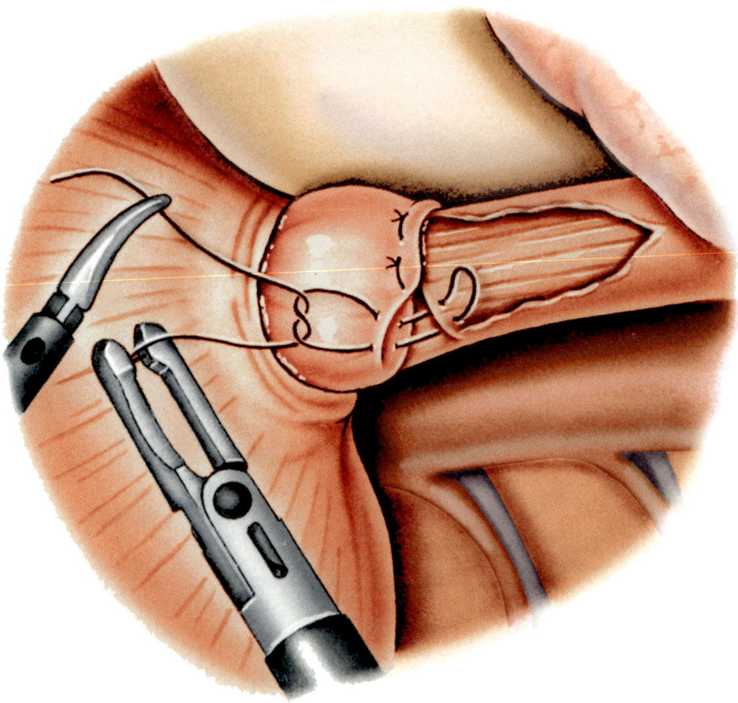

Figure IIIE-6,G: With the posterior sutures across the hiatus left untied, the first row of three sutures between the fundus and the esophagus is completed. For the purpose of clear illustration, they are shown at 6, 9, and 12 o'clock—ideally, they should be at 1 o'clock anteriorly and at 5 o'clock posteriorly.

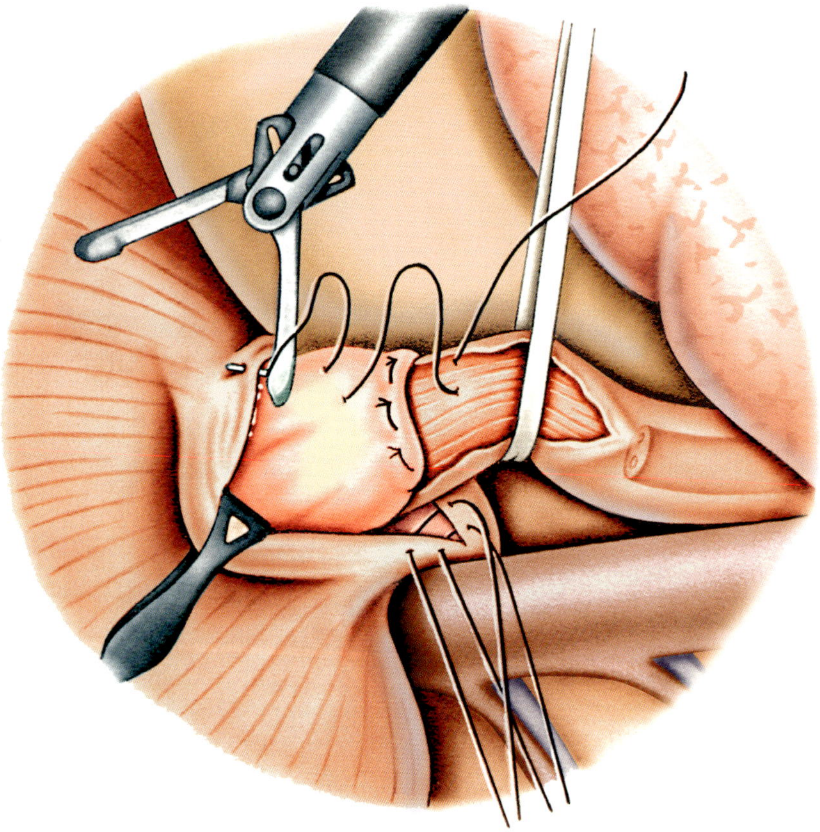

Figure IIIE-6,H: A second row of three mattress sutures is placed between the esophagus, gastric fundus, and fibrous rim of the diaphragm. The posterior sutures across the hiatus remain untied. The esophagoscope "lurks" proximally and is used to indicate the exact gastroesophageal junction, which it is often difficult to define from the outside in patients who have had longstanding reflux and esophageal shortening of some degree. It is also used to measure the intraluminal length of the repair, which should be at least 4 cm.

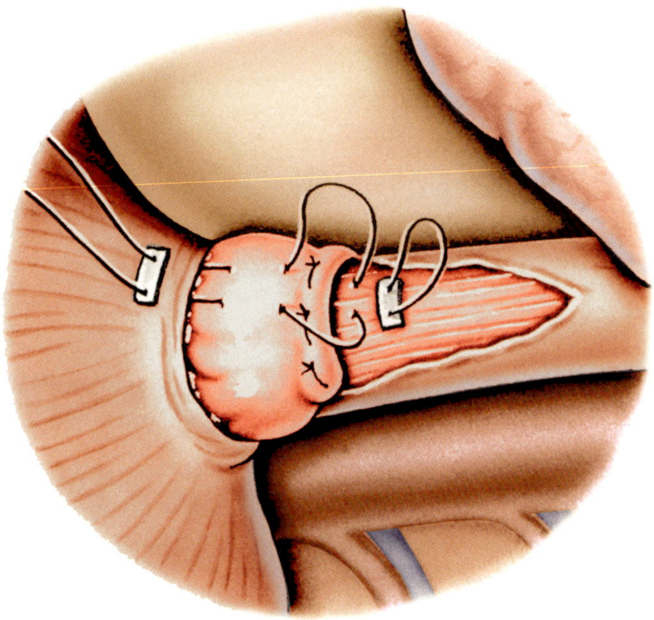

Figure IIIE-6,I: As for the first row of sutures, the second row may be placed over pledgets to protect and hold the placement of these sutures since they will be under considerable stress from diaphragmatic and esophageal motion, often going in opposite directions during deglutition, hiccups, and vomiting.

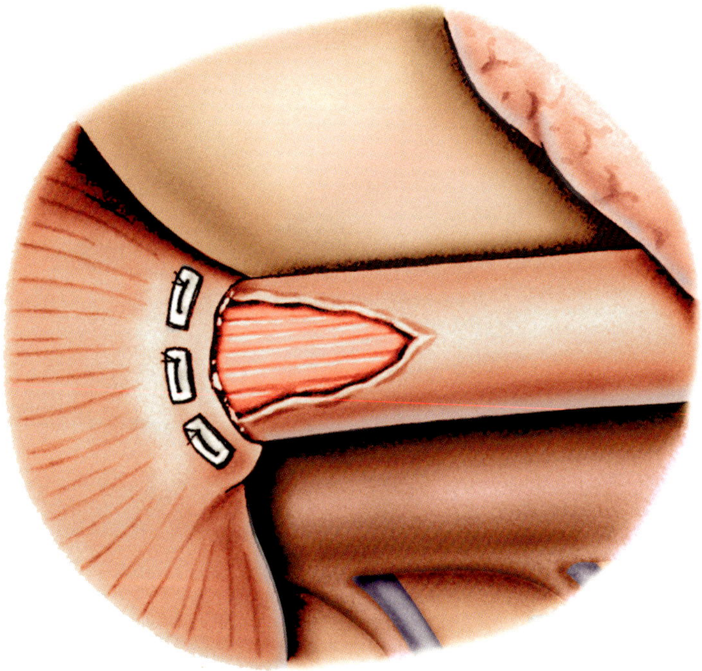

Figure III E-6,J: As the second row of sutures is tied, the collar—consisting of vertically invaginated esophagus (4 cm) into the gastric fundus over its anterior-lateral-posterior, two-thirds circumference and representing the repair—is repositioned into the abdomen and anchored to the peritoneal surface of the hiatus. The sutures closing the hiatus posteriorly are now tied with the esophagoscope or a bougie in place. As for the first row, the second row sutures should ideally be placed at 1, 9, and 5 o'clock.

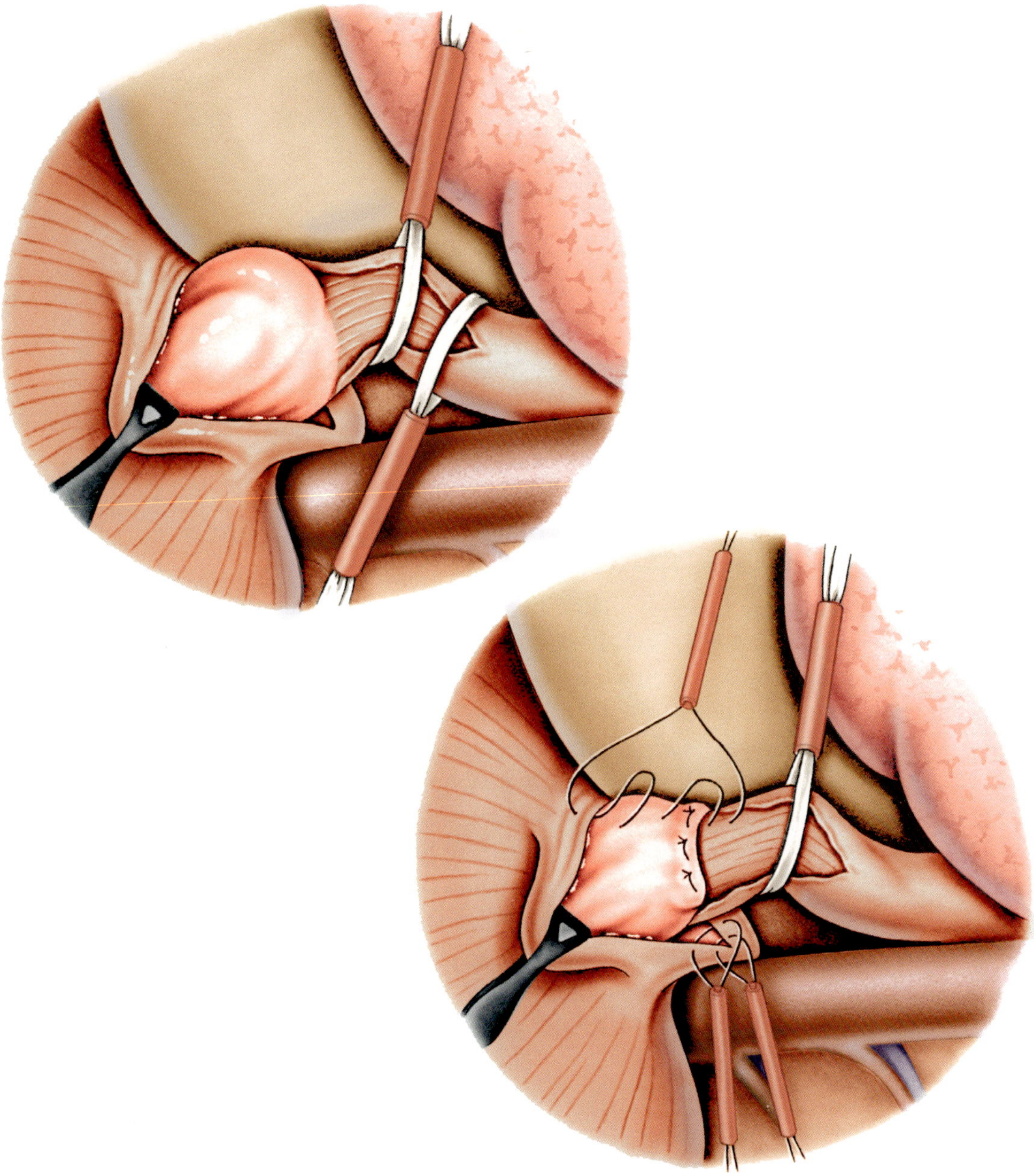

Figure IIIE-6,K,L: During this procedure, the tape to elevate the esophagus and the many sutures remaining temporarily untied may create a confusing jungle in a rather confined space. We have found it helpful to sheathe each pair of strings left untied, with individual red rubber catheters, to avoid time-consuming sorting out and interference with dissecting and suturing instruments.

NISSEN FUNDOPLICATION

When persistent gastroesophageal reflux can not be effectively controlled by nonoperative treatment such as pills, potions, and dietary changes, a Nissen fundoplication offers remedial action and represents the first choice approach for the patient whose left upper quadrant and epigastrium have remained untouched by a surgical procedure and hence are free of adhesions. If there has been longstanding esophagitis and shortening of the esophagus, the simple wrap of a flap of gastric fundus around the esophagus may not be possible. In these patients, the Collis gastroplasty, lengthening the esophagus with a gastric tube of the lesser curvature in continuity, and a modified Nissen fundoplication of the remaining fundus and greater curvature "dog ear" will accomplish the same result as a single fundoplication (Figure III-21, A to G). Both operations can be performed by laparotomy and laparoscopy. In all patients, a preliminary esophagoscopy with four quadrant biopsies of the lower esophageal segment should have established the fact that there is no malignant transformation associated with longstanding esophagitis.

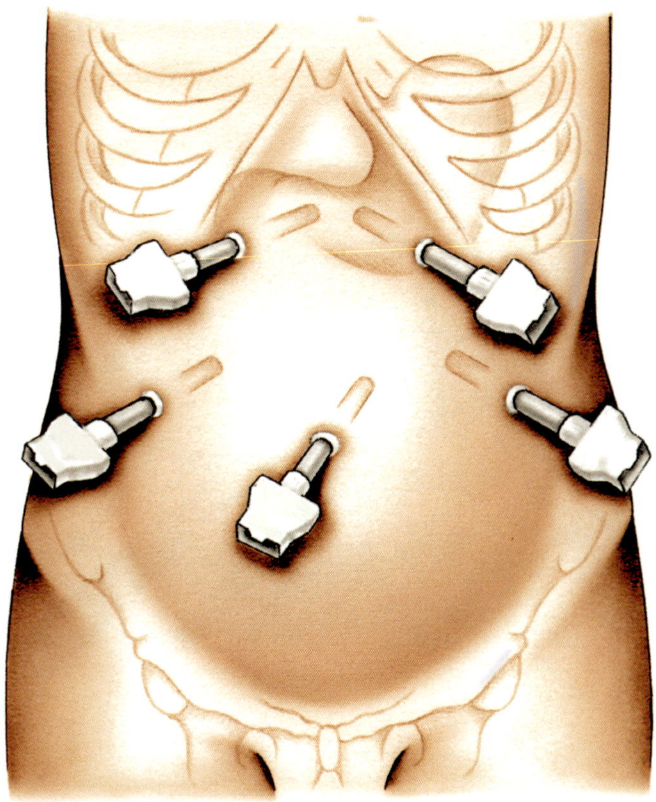

Figure IIIE-7,A: The approach is usually through five ports: the umbilical trocar for the placement of the laparoscope, two trocar sites on each side of the epigastrium close to the mid-costal margins, and two sites in the right and left mid-abdominal areas at the borders between upper and lower quadrants.

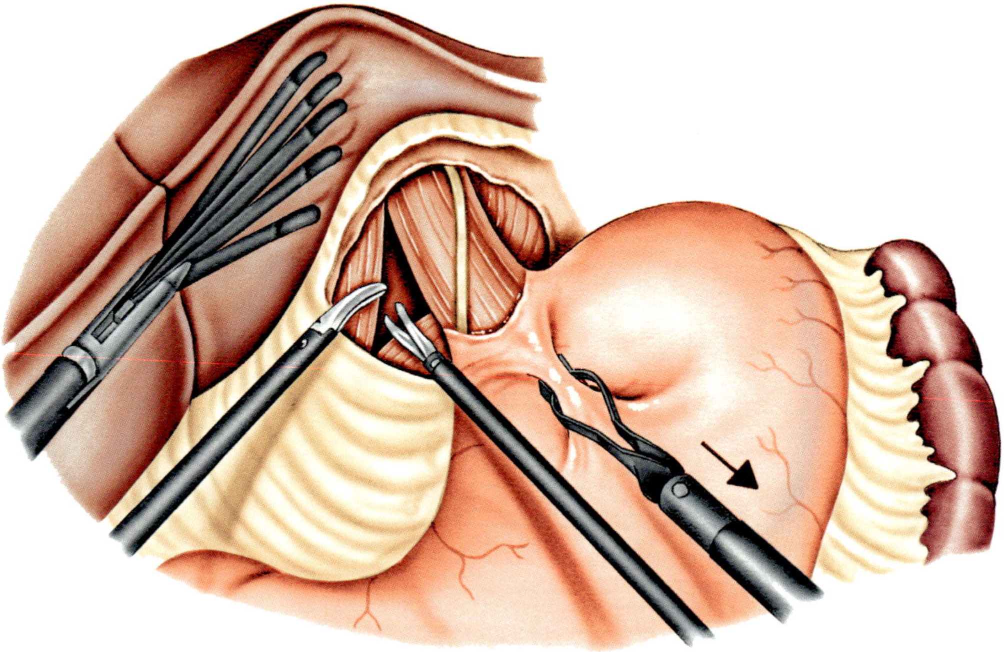

Figure IIIE-7,B: The left lobe of the liver is elevated with a sturdy fan retractor introduced through the right epigastric port. Although incision of the triangular ligament is occasionally required to facilitate this retraction, it is not undertaken on a routine basis because of occasional bothersome oozing of blood from that site. With gentle traction on the fundus of the stomach and on the esophagus, short gastric vessels along the upper reaches of the greater curvature and branches from the left gastric vessels along the lesser curvature are coagulated and divided to lend greater mobility to the GE junction. The areolar tissue around the hiatus is dissected and the phrenoesophageal ligament is incised, to expose the GE junction and the pillars of the diaphragmatic crus.

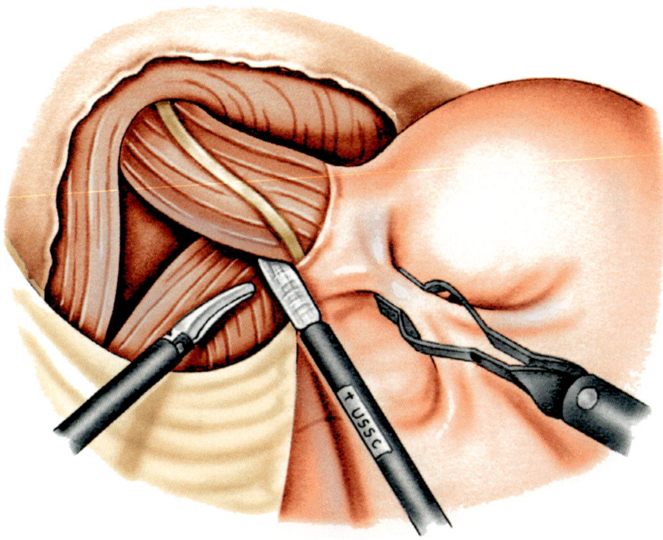

Figure IIIE-7,C: With continued traction to the left, on the anterior wall of the stomach below the GE junction, the abdominal esophageal segment is liberated in its entire circumference, starting from behind the junction upward into the mediastinum. The vagus nerves are identified and preserved during this dissection. By delineating the esophagus at its junction with the stomach, it is easier to keep the upward dissection close to the circumference of the esophageal tube and avoid injury to the left pleura by an "errant" scissors tip.

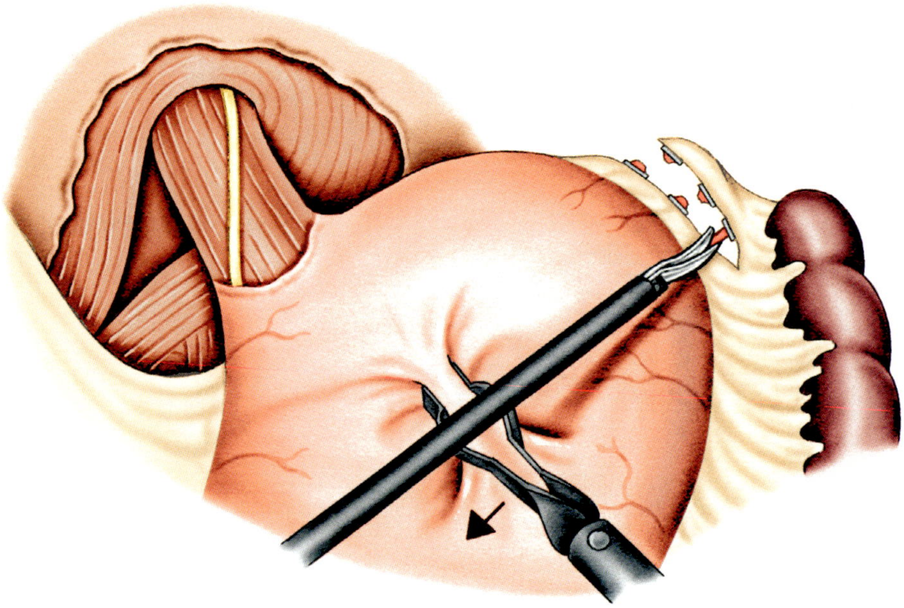

Figure IIIE-7,D: In order to give full mobility to the fundus along the descending portion of the greater curvature, it may be necessary to divide three or four additional short gastric vessels, while taking great care to protect the spleen, which is usually pushed posteriorly by the pneumoperitoneum.

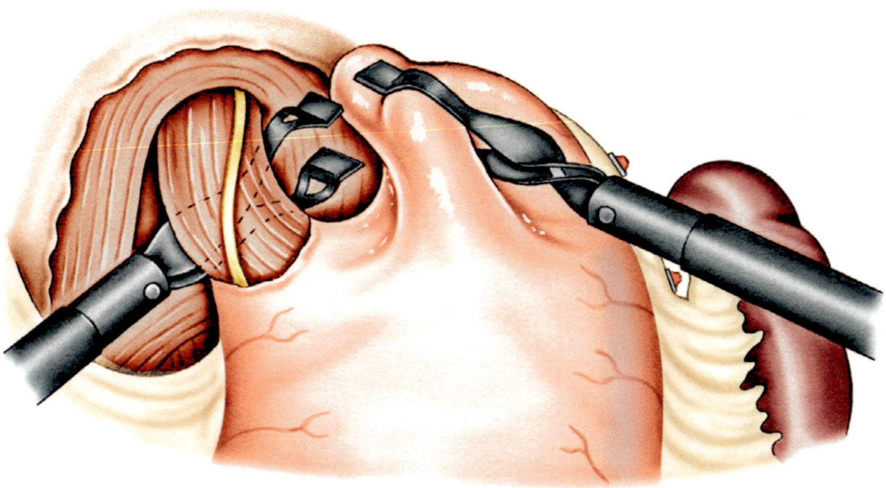

Figure IIIE-7,E: A Babcock clamp is passed behind the fully liberated esophagus, anterior to the left crural pillar. The wall of the fundus is elevated with a second Babcock clamp at a point on the fundus and apex of the greater curvature that is mobile and of sufficient length to pass behind the esophagus and wrap around its right side.

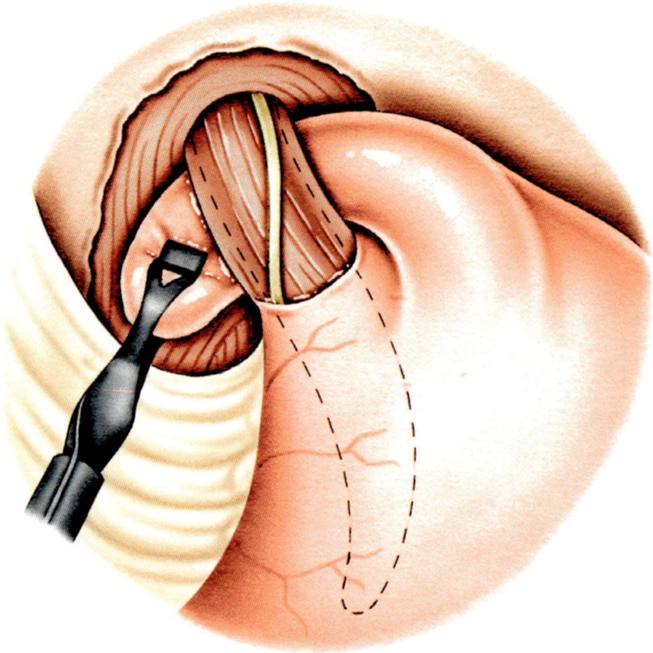

Figure IIIE-7,F: The future collar of fundus is grasped with the right-sided Babcock clamp and pulled behind the esophagus to the right anterior aspect of the GE junction. A large intraluminal bougie is advanced.

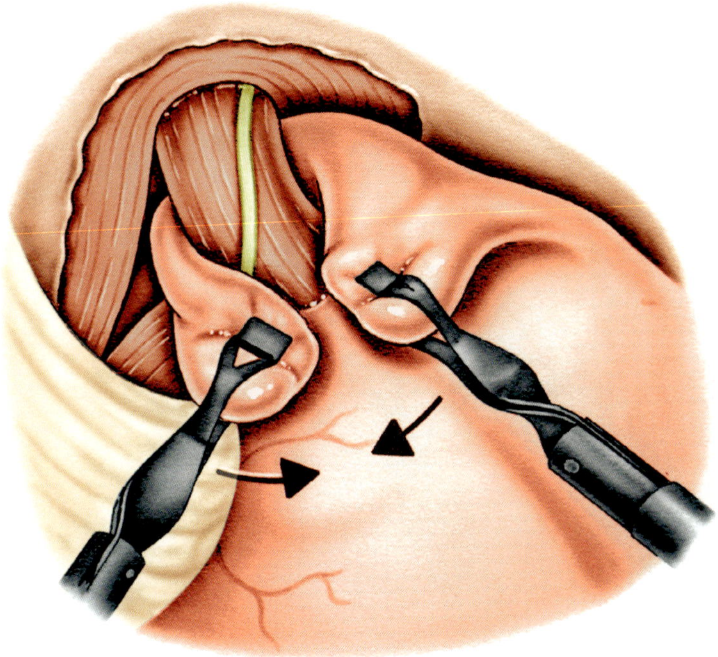

Figure IIIE-7,G: The remaining left side of the fundus is elevated by a second Babcock clamp to meet with its right counterpart over the GE junction that is calibrated by the intraluminal bougie. This encounter serves in the appreciation of any number of parameters, for example, loose vs tight collar, unsatisfactory mobility of the wrap, insufficient height of the collar to ensure a safe placement of the sutures and to forecast a reliable functional result. All of these factors can be evaluated and corrected before the final step of closing the collar anteriorly.

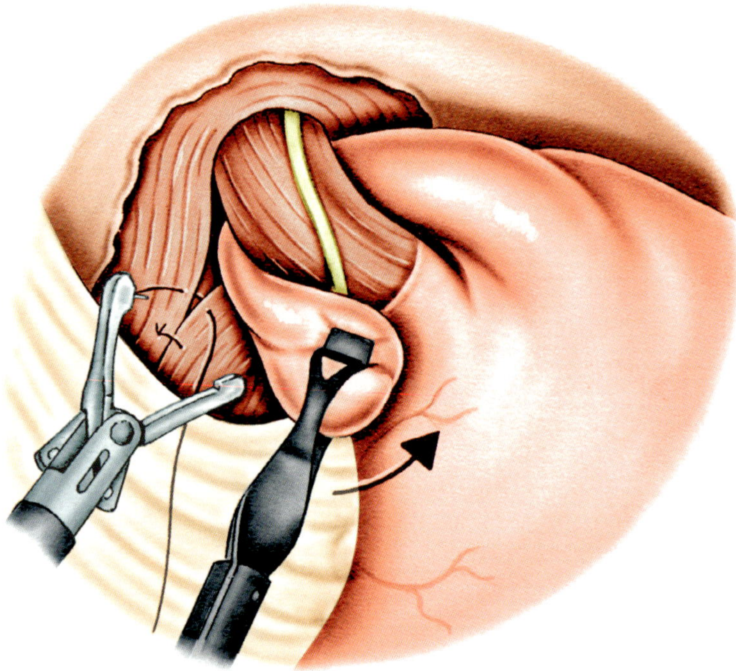

Figure IIIE-7,H: With the right side of the collar held out of the way, on gentle traction to elevate the esophagus, the hiatus is repaired deep to the fundic flap with two to three sutures placed and tied with the previously mentioned intraluminal bougie in place.

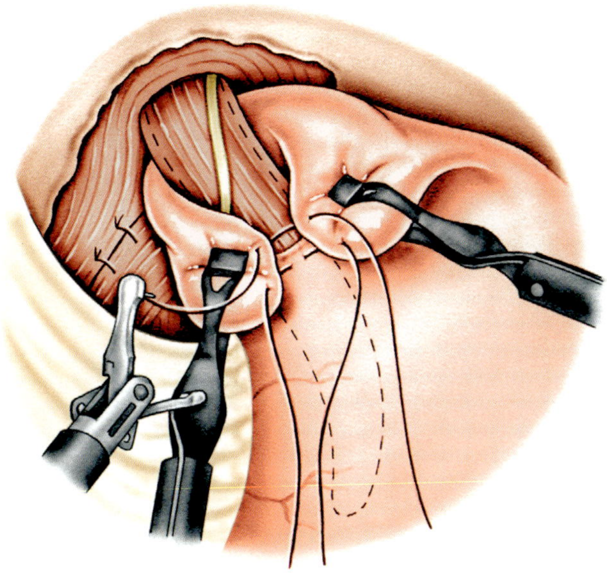

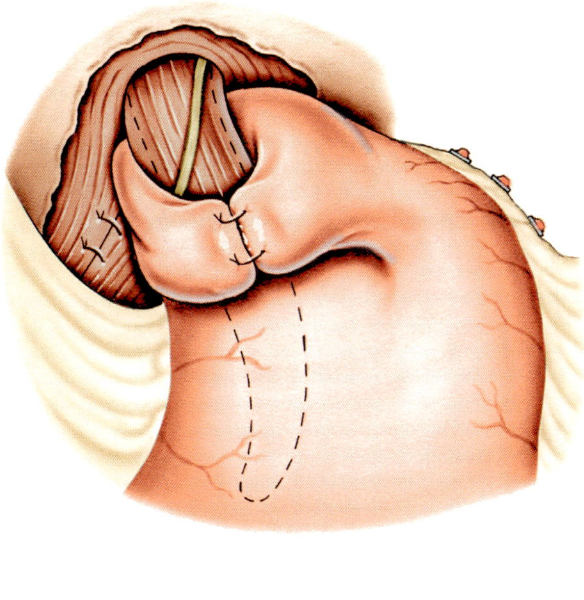

Figure IIIE-7,I: All that remains to be done is to close the collar anteriorly with two or three sutures. In order to prevent slippage of the collar into the mediastinum, the lower-most closing suture is taken through the anterior gastric wall, just below the GE junction.

Figure IIIE-7,J: A floppy wrap is obtained, with sutures tied over the bougie.

PORTOAZYGOUS DISCONNECTION

Portoazygos disconnection is an alternative method in the treatment of bleeding esophageal varices that can be accomplished by laparoscopic means, employing the technique described in Figure III-22, F and G. While the TIPS procedure in the emergency treatment of bleeding esophageal varices has gained great acceptance in specialized centers, it does require appropriate staff with expertise in interventional radiology equipment adapted to this special task. In hospitals that receive the occasional patient with variceal bleeding and that are faced with the responsibility to undertake a life-saving operation, portoazygous disconnection represents an acceptable alternative approach to TIPS, especially since it can be done by laparotomy and laparoscopy. Both the TIPS and portoazygous disconnection procedures are valuable as temporizing salvage operations in patients who are candidates for liver transplantation, since they do not alter the anatomy of the portal vein or of the inferior vena cava.

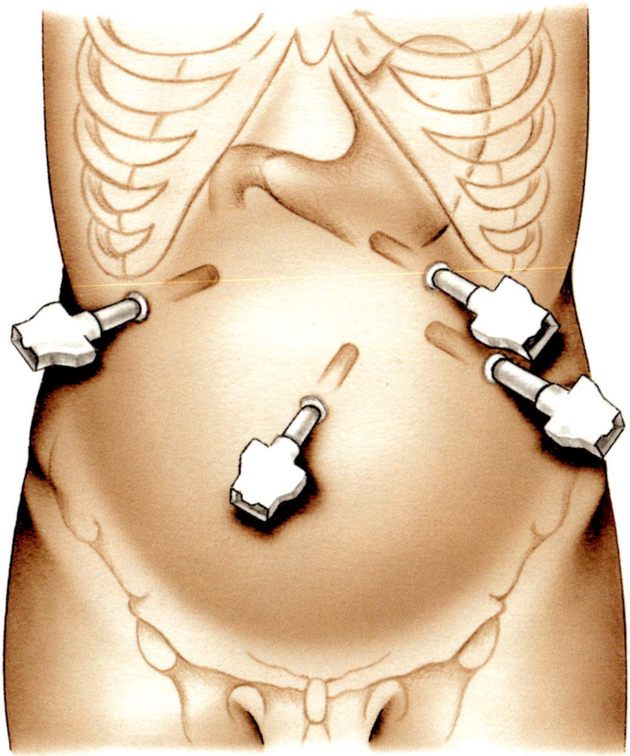

Figure IIIE-8,A: Port placements are established at the umbilicus for the laparoscope, at the left midclavicular line at the level of the umbilicus, below the left midcostal margin, and at the right midclavicular line below the costal margin.

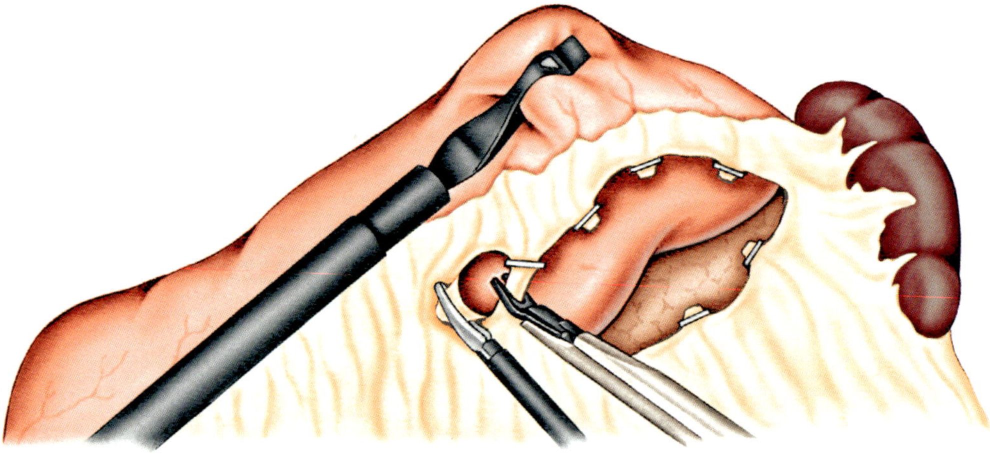

Figure IIIE-8,B: The greater curvature of the stomach is elevated with a Babcock clamp, and the lesser sac is entered by dividing the gastroepiploic vessels between clips.

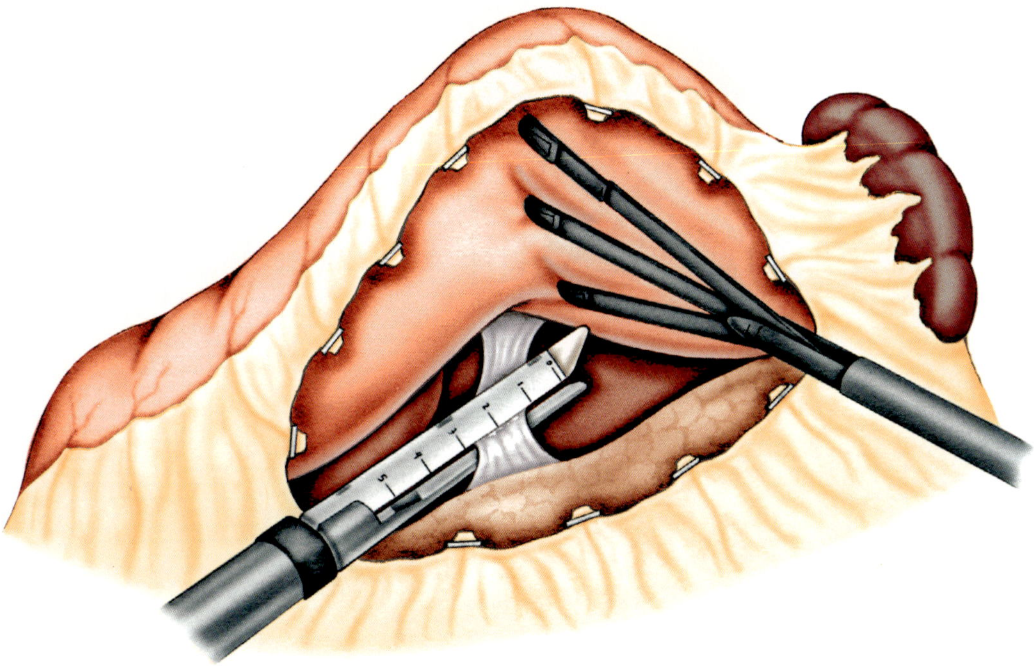

Figure IIIE-8,C: The posterior wall of the stomach is elevated with a fan retractor. The gastropancreatic fold is identified and transected between two triple rows of staples with the ENDO GIA stapler.

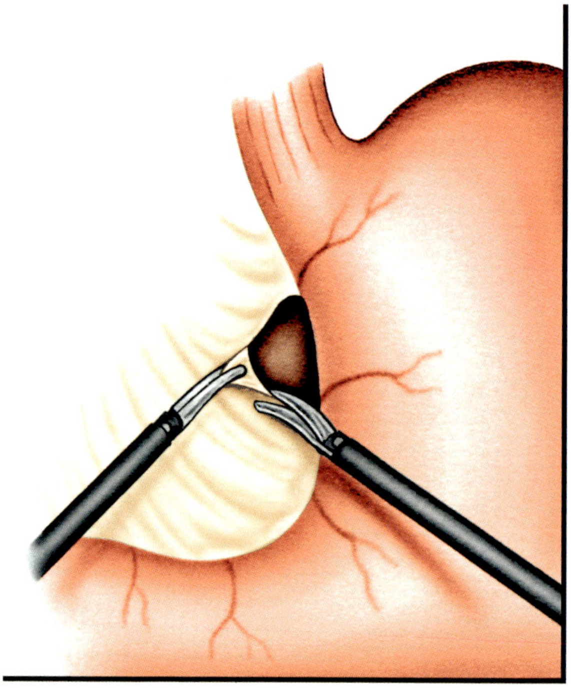

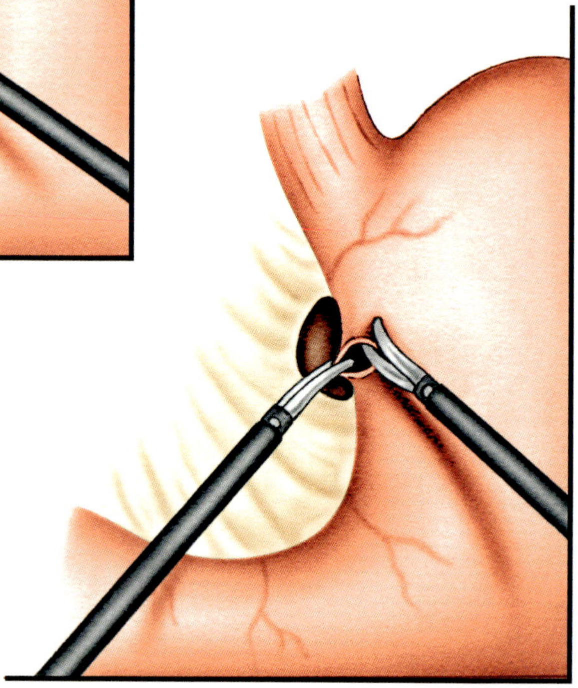

Figure IIIE-8,D: With the stomach pulled down and to the left with a Babcock clamp and the left lobe of the liver elevated with a fan retractor, the gastrohepatic ligament is incised just distal to the GE junction and the lesser sac is entered.

Figure IIIE-8,E: The lesser curvature is incised, high on the stomach, barely caudal to the junction, to accommodate the anvil of the stapler.

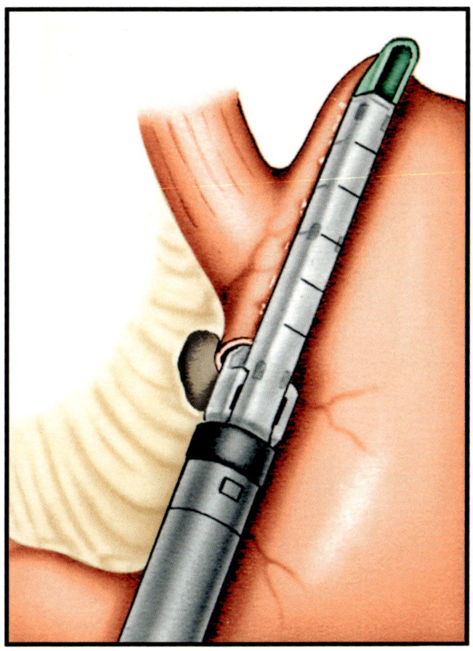

Figure IIIE-8,F: The anvil of the ENDO TA 30 instrument for a narrow GE junction or the ENDO GIA 60 instrument with a SGIA cartridge for a wide GE junction is inserted into the lumen of the stomach and directed anteriorly toward the angle of His. The cartridge of the instrument is on the serosal surface, holding the anterior wall of the stomach between the anvil and cartridge. The instrument is closed and activated, placing three or six rows of hemostatic staples respectively on the anterior wall of the stomach.

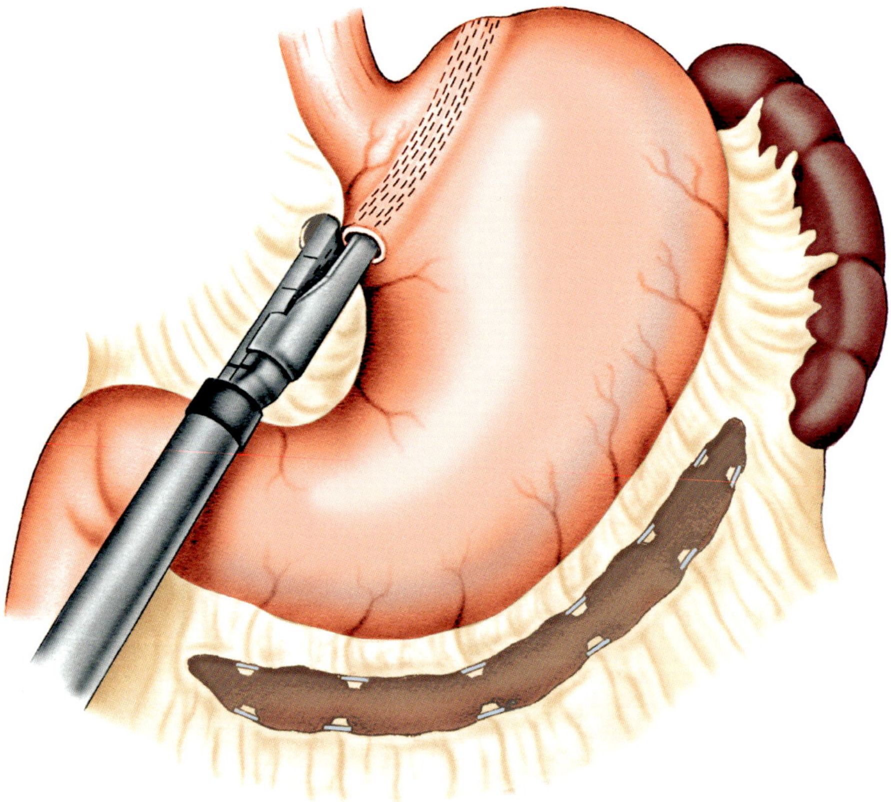

Figure IIIE-8,G: The instrument is reloaded and reapplied posteriorly, holding the posterior gastric wall between intraluminal anvil and exterior cartridge. Closing and activating the instrument completes the circle of staples around the gastric side of the GE junction.

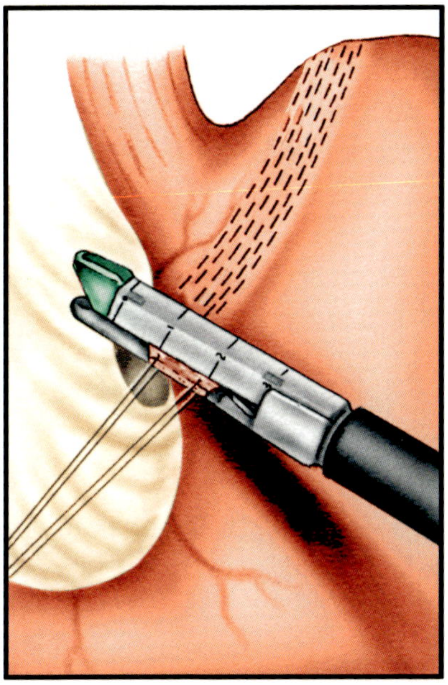

Figure IIIE-8,H: Stay sutures are placed at each end of the gastrotomy and are put on traction to elevate the pouting borders of the gastric opening. The ENDO TA 30 or ENDO GIA 30 instrument is used to close the gastrotomy wound.

SUGGESTED READING

Akiyama H. *Surgery for Cancer of the Esophagus*. Baltimore, Md: Williams & Wilkins; 1990.

Akiyama H, Tsurumaru M. Stapling in esophageal resections. In: *Current Practice of Surgical Stapling*. Philadelphia, Pa: Lea & Febiger; 1991.

Behl PR, Holden MP, Brown AH. Three years' experience with esophageal stapling device. *Ann Surg.* 1983;198:134-136.

Collard JM, Otte JB, Reynaert M, Kestens PJ. Long gastroplasties with the GIA stapler in esophageal surgery. In: *Current Practice of Surgical Stapling*. Philadelphia, Pa: Lea & Febiger; 1991.

Dei Poli M, Gasparri G, Casalegno PA, et al. Mechanical sutures in esophageal surgery [in Italian]. *Minerva Chir.* 1991;46:1229-1233.

Dickson GH. Some clinical and technical aspects of circular stapled anastomoses of rectum and oesophagus. *Ann R Coll Surg Engl.* 1989;71:59-63.

Diviacco P, Danovaro L, Molinello P, et al. Original method of the treatment of achalasic megaesophagus with EEA stapler [in Italian]. *G Chir.* 1991;12:515-519.

Donnelly RJ, Kaplan D, Whyte RI, Muehrcke DD. Esophago-gastrectomy using the EEA stapler. In: *Current Practice of Surgical Stapling*. Philadelphia, Pa: Lea & Febiger; 1991.

Dorsey JS, Esses S, Goldberg M, Stone R. Esophagogastrectomy using the auto suture EEA surgical stapling instrument. *Ann Thorac Surg.* 1980;30:308-312.

Fasching W. The double stapling technic of the esophagus. Mechanical esophagojejunostomy without purse-string suture [in German]. *Chirurg.* 1989;60:301-302.

Fasching W, Moritz E. Circular staple anastomoses in the gastrointestinal tract with the staplers SPTU and EEA [in German]. *Chirurg.* 1980; 51:644-650.

Fatsis ME, Hatzinis AC, Antypas GD. Automatic stapling devices in the surgical treatment of esophageal diverticula. *Scand J Thorac Cardiovasc Surg.* 1991;25:195-197.

Fekete F, Gayet B, Place S, Biagini J. Four hundred esophageal anastomoses with a stapler. *Int Surg.* 1989;74:69-72.

Fekete F, Sauvanet A, Belghiti J. Results of 1000 esophageal resections with stapled anastomoses. In: *Minimally Invasive Surgery and New Technology*. St. Louis, Mo: Quality Medical Publishing; 1994.

Gayet B. Total or partial esophageal replacement or bypass for benign conditions of the esophagus. In: *Current Practice of Surgical Stapling*. Philadelphia, Pa: Lea & Febiger; 1991.

Giraud RM, Berzin SA. Reversed gastric esophagoplasty. *Surg Ann*. 1990;22:263-279.

Griffen WO Jr. Stapling in gastroesophageal surgery. *Surg Clin North Am*. 1984;64:529-542.

Hopkins RA, Alexander JC, Postlethwait RW. Stapled esophagogastric anastomosis. *Am J Surg*. 1984;147:283-287.

Huang XM. Stapled anastomoses in esophageal resections. In: *Current Practice of Surgical Stapling*. Philadephia, Pa: Lea & Febiger; 1991.

Humphrey EW. Stapling techniques in esophageal replacement. *Surg Clin North Am*. 1984;64:499-510.

Imamura M, Ohishi K, Tobe T. Retrosternal esophagogastrostomy with the EEA stapler. *Surg Gynecol Obstet*. 1987;164:368-371.

Kaplan DK, Whyte RI, Donnelly RJ. Oesophagogastrectomy using stapling instruments. *Eur J Cardiothorac Surg*. 1988;2:95-99.

Kivelitz H, Ulrich B. Mechanical sutures in esophageal surgery [in German]. *Langenbecks Arch Chir*. 1981;355:455-457.

Kockel N, Ulrich B. Anastomosis of the cervical esophagus to a greater curvature isoperistaltic tube or colon segment with stapling instruments. In: *Current Practice of Surgical Stapling*. Philadelphia, Pa: Lea & Febiger; 1991.

Kockel N, Ulrich B. Trans-hiatal resection for carcinoma of the distal esophagus and esophagogastric junction: esophagogastrostomy and esophago-jejunostomy with manual and mechanical sutures. In: *Current Practice of Surgical Stapling*. Philadelphia, Pa: Lea & Febiger; 1991.

Kuster GGR. The value of an indwelling tube through a stapled esophageal anastomosis. In: *Current Practice of Surgical Stapling*. Philadelphia, Pa: Lea & Febiger; 1991.

Legaspi A, Irani H. Stapled transabdominal lower esophageal anastomosis without purse-string suture. *Surg Gynecol Obstet*. 1990;170:156-158.

Lersmacher J, Kantartzis M, Hoffmann E. Removal of Zenker's diverticula using automatic staplers [in German]. *Chirurg*. 1989;60:163-167.

Mathisen DJ, Grillo HC, Wilkins EW Jr, Moncure AC, Hilgenberg AD. Transthoracic esophagectomy: a safe approach to carcinoma of the esophagus. *Ann Thorac Surg*. 1988;45: 137-143.

McManus KG, Ritchie AJ, McGuigan J, Stevenson HM. Gibbons JR. Sutures, staplers, leaks and strictures. A review of anastomoses in oesophageal resection at Royal Victoria Hospital, Belfast 1977-1986. *Eur J Cardiothorac Surg*. 1990;4:97-100.

Misumi A, Misumi K, Harada K, Murakami A, Kondo H, Akagi M. Transabdominal operation for carcinoma of the gastric cardia: application of pulling-up retractor and EEA stapler. *Int Surg*. 1989; 74:223-228.

Muehrcke DD, Donnelly RJ. Complications after esophagogastrectomy using stapling instruments. *Ann Thorac Surg*. 1989;48:257-262.

Page RD, Khalil JF, Whyte RI, Kaplan DK, Donnelly RJ. Esophagogastrectomy via left thoracophrenotomy. *Ann Thorac Surg*. 1990;49:763-766.

Paramo JC, Summerall J, Poppiti R, Mesko ThW. Validation of sentinel node mapping in patients with colon cancer. *Ann Surg Oncol*. 2002;9(6):550-554.

Park KG, Munro A. Simple solution to the short oesophagus encountered at abdominal fundoplication. *Br J Surg*. 1992;79:51.

Shahinian TK, Bowen JR, Dorman BA, Soderberg CH Jr, Thompson WR. Experience with EEA stapling device. *Am J Surg*. 1980;139:549-553.

Spina GP, Rosati R, Rebuffat C, Montorsi M, Zago M. The EEA circular mechanical stapler in digestive surgery. Analysis of 76 cases [in Italian]. *Minerva Chir*. 1984;39:197-203.

Steichen FM. Abdominal approach to the Collis gastroplasty and Nissen fundoplication. *Surg Gynecol Obstet*. 1986;162:272-274.

Steichen FM. Varieties of stapled anastomoses of the esophagus. *Surg Clin North Am*. 1984;64:481-498.

Steichen FM, Dibbins AW, Weiner ES. *Recent Advances in Paediatric Surgery*. 3rd ed. New York, NY: Churchill Livingstone; 1975.

Steichen FM, Ravitch MM. *Stapling in Surgery*. Chicago, Ill: Year Book Medical Publishers; 1984.

Sugimachi K, Ikeda M, Ueo H, Kai H, Okudaira Y, Inokuchi K. Clinical efficacy of the stapled anastomosis in esophageal reconstruction. *Ann Thorac Surg*. 1982;33:374-378.

Sugimachi K, Ohno S, Maekawa S, Mori M, Kuwano H, Ueo H. Safety of EEA staplers for anastomosis between upper esophagus and the gastric tube. *J Surg Oncol*. 1990;43:40-44.

Talmi YP, Finkelstein Y, Sadov R, Shvili RY, Zohar Y. Use of a linear stapler in excision of Zenker's diverticulum. *Head Neck*. 1989;11:150-152.

Taylor TV, Knox RA, Pullan BR. Vertical gastric plication: an operation for gastro-oesophageal reflux. *Ann R Coll Surg Engl*. 1989;71:31-36.

Wahl W, Junginger T, Bottger T. Surgical stapler technique for gastric tube formation and anastomosis after esophageal resection [in German]. *Langenbecks Arch Chir*. 1992;377:107-111.

West PN, Marbarger JP, Martz MN, Roper CL. Esophagogastrostomy with the EEA stapler. *Ann Surg*. 1981;193:76-81.

Wetstejn L, Kirby DF, Shubert ML, Ali MM. Proximal stapled esophagogastric anastomosis. *South Med J*. 1988;81:279-280.

Wilson SE, Stone R, Scully M, Ozeran L, Benfield JR. Modern management of anastomotic leak after esophagogastrectomy. *Am J Surg*. 1982;144:95-101.

Wong J, Cheung H, Lui R, Fan YW, Smith A, Siu KF. Esophagogastric anastomosis performed with a stapler: the occurrence of leakage and stricture. *Surgery*. 1987;101:408-415.

Woods SD, McGuire LJ, Chung SC, Crofts TJ, Li AK. Intrathoracic stapled anastomosis after oesophagectomy for cancer. *Aust N Z J Surg*. 1989;59:647-651.

INDEX

F

G

H

I

J

K

L

M

N

P